T0171328

Ju-Jutsu

A COMPREHENSIVE GUIDE

James Moclair

authorHOUSE®

AuthorHouse™ UK Ltd.
500 Avebury Boulevard
Central Milton Keynes, MK9 2BE
www.authorhouse.co.uk
Phone: 08001974150

First published by AuthorHouse 8/13/2009

ISBN: 978-1-4490-0776-8 (sc)

This book is printed on acid-free paper.

Books by James Moclair

A Breath of Fresh Air, Kempo Karate Novice to Intermediate

ISBN 9781425930295

Paperback (8..25 x 11)

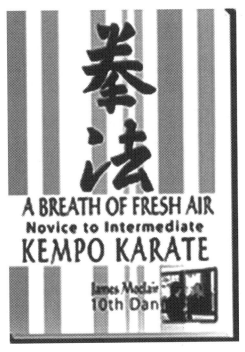

A journey starts with the first step and your martial arts career starts when you first step into a Dojo (martial arts training hall). My book will help people of all ages who have never done any karate before to understand the basic techniques with step by step guidance and take you on an exiting journey from novice to intermediate level. More importantly you will learn a comprehensive range of practical self defence routines that are simple to follow.

Even if you have practiced another style of karate or other martial art you will, with the easy to follow photographic illustrations be able to gain new and sometimes quite unique skills quite quickly and that will be of great benefit to your own martial arts

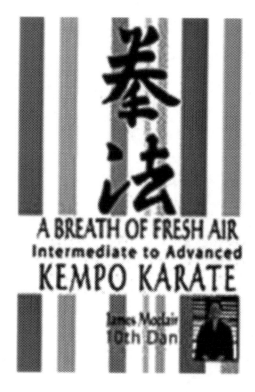

A BREATH OF FRESH AIR
Intermediate to Advanced
KEMPO KARATE

James Macbir
10th Dan

After the success of James's first book, Kempo Karate, novice to intermediate, the martial art world has waited in eagerness for his next book.

The wait is now over, in this second edition, Kempo karate, intermediate to advanced, the author has once again shown that he is a true master of the art of kempo karate by explaining in explicit detail the intricacies of techniques that have eluded many martial artist's.

What is even more amazing is that James has taken the ideology and concepts on the fascinating martial art and added his own martial experience to it to create a style that is unique to him. The system is a self defence martial art and deals with realistic attacks that are happening every day, on every street around the world!

Each technique throughout this book flows in a natural martial manner. Add to this the easy to follow photographic illustrations and vividly written explanations and what the reader will get is a visual and mental self-assurance that will inspire them to try these techniques out in there own martial arts club.

What is even more beneficial to the reader is that once you have tried, practised and mastered these techniques, you will have the ability to defend yourself against some extreme attacks. Now that is life saving and has to be priceless!

Even if you yourself are an experienced martial artist, from a completely different martial background, this book will also benefit you. Some of the author's techniques are practical but absolutely unique, why not utilize and adapt them in with your own art or style; you have nothing to lose and some fantastic self defence concepts to gain.

About the Author

This is the third martial arts book written by James Moclair, he has a life times experience in martial arts and is a Professor of Bu-Jutsu, (Japanese martial arts). James teaches his martial arts professionally and has been doing this since 1979. At this point of time James has been training in the martial arts for over forty five years.

James has an impressive martial arts career that has taken him around the world and has even been World Ju-Jutsu Demonstration Champion and Gold medallist representing England at the World Ju-Jutsu Games 1986.

Also in 1986 James Moclair took the British martial arts community by storm by also becoming the British Nunchacku Champion and even today he is still considered to be one of the finest nunchaku practitioners in the world. James has his own web site dedicated to the nunchaku, it is: http://www.freewebs.com/nunchaku.

James Moclair's current martial arts grades are; Soke Shodai 1st generation founder of Eikokyu-Ryu Tai Jutsu Renmei martial arts systems, 10th Dan Ju-jutsu.

He also holds additional grades as follow's arts;

- 8th Dan Kempo Karate.

- 8th Dan Ko-Budo.

- 6th Dan Aiki-jutsu.

- 5th Dan Traditional Judo, 5thDan Combat Judo and Combat Ki Master.

- 5th Dan -Godan in the style of Senai Seisshinryu Shihandokai Karate-Do Jutsu.

- 8th Dan / Hachidan "Master" Shoshin Goshin Jutsu.

- James also holds many other dan grades in other arts and styles.

James's martial arts grades are recognised by numerous associations around the world and include the distinguished ALL JAPAN JU-JITSU INTERNATIONAL FEDERATION, Martial Arts Association- International, International Board of Black Belts, The World Organizer of Martial Arts INC. USA, WOMA International Council For Higher Martial Arts Science Edudcation INC. World Ju-Jutsu / Aiki - Bujutsu Federation, Australian Ju-Jutsu Federation Incorporated and Bushi Kai International and many, many other eminent world class organisations.

James is the founder of the Eikokyu-Ryu Tai Jutsu Renmei. The ryu is broken down into Ju-Jutsu, Kempo Karate, Aiki-Jutsu, Ko-Budo, Combat Judo and Combat Ki.

The Eikokyu-Ryu Tai Jutsu Renmei is recognised as a legitimate martial arts system with James Moclair as its founder by;

Bushi Kai International,

INTERNATIONAL SOKE-HEAD FOUNDER SOCIETY KOKUSAI SOKE-SHUSO KAI HOMBU INTERNATIONAL SOKE SHIP,

HEAD FOUNDER, HEAD FAMILIES, GRANDMASTERS COUNCIL.

World Hombu Budo / Bugei Kokusai Renmie MMA-I, International Board of Black Belts,

The World Organizer of Martial Arts INC. USA.

WOMA International Council For Higher Martial Arts Science Education INC,

United Sokeship Alliance International

Soke Menkyo Kai.

World Head Master Council of Martial Arts. HEADMASTERS / HEAD FAMILY UNDER THE SAIGO HA DAITO RYU RENGOKAI LINEAGE.

Martial Arts Association- International.

The World Jug Tai Association, Office of International Affairs & the Division of Martial Arts Centre for Martial Arts Research.

Each of the above has bestowed the title of;

Soke Shodai, First Generation Founder to James Moclair.

In 2007, the Fighting Arts Brotherhood Hall of Fame inducted James Moclair for his contribution to the growth of Martial Arts World Wide and also awarded him "Founder of the Year 2007"

James is recognised as a "Grandmaster" by the International Board of Black Belts, World Grand Master's Union and the World Black Belt Council and "Honourable Grandmaster" by the International Grandmaster Committee & World Ambassador Council, International Council of Higher Martial Arts Education and World Head Master Council of Martial Arts. In 2009, the World Grand Master's Union appointed Professor James Moclair as its Official Representative for England.

Over the years James has set up several martial arts organisations and he is the founder and President of Bushi Kai International, The founder and President of the Guild of Professional Martial Artist's.

James also hold key positions in numerous organisations, some of which are listed below;

European Vice President to the Soke Menkyo Kai

http://www.freewebs.com/soke-menkyo-kai-europe

United Kingdom Coordinator to the World Organisation of Self Defence www.wosd.org

Official J.F.C Federation Representative for England.

N.V.Q Martial Arts Consortium Centre Head with Royal Society of Arts.

President of the Martial Arts Olympic Committee Organization for England

Eikoku-Ryu Tai Jutsu Renmei Representative for England for ChunJiDo International

Intercontinental Director for England to the Intercontinental Martial Arts Union.

Recently James joined the ranks of the elite, 'THE WORLD MARTIAL ARTS FRIENDSHIP SOCIETY' and is recognised in the World Masters directory.

You can find a current listing of James's grades and achievements by visiting the following web site: http://www.taijutsukwai.com

I think you will agree that James's achievements are outstanding, however this has only come about by years of dedication and hard work.

James's life evolves around his martial arts, he spends over seventy six hours a week at his Dojo, (martial arts centre) where he teaches, writes his books and keeps up his own martial arts practice. And if you think that is impressive let me tell you that he also does this seven days a week!

Contents

Ju-Jutsu A comprehensive guide

By James Moclair Soke Shodai 10th Dan

The young boy walked into the local school lobby and asked the elderly gentle man who was busy mopping the floor, "Excuse me Sir, where are the Ju-Jutsu classes being held?" The old man looked hard at the boy and said, "Get the hell out of here son, the classes are for adults only! Kids aren't allowed in the school in the evenings! The boy in a polite voice said "Sir, I know that they are adult classes but I am a student of Judo and I was hoping to have a word with the club Sensei" "The what?" the old man hissed back. "Sir, Sensei means teacher" the boy informed the now irate old man. The old man turned his back on the boy, swilled his mop in the bucket and said "There in the gym, down the hall, first on your left" he then turned, glared at the boy and said, "don't walk on my clean floor!" The boy politely thanked the old man and made his way to the gym.

As the boy approached the gym he noticed that the double gym doors were ajar and he could see that a small number of people were warming up on the Tatami, (mat area). As a sign of respect the boy stood at the door entrance, removed his shoes and made a small bow. He could see the Sensei (Teacher) was busy instructing the class students and it is customary in a Dojo that you never interrupt the Sensei (teacher) until he is ready to speak to you, so the boy just stood and patiently waited.

The Sensei (teacher) was a slim man, clean shaven and in his mid forties. He was of average height and was wearing an immaculate white Gi (martial arts suit). To hold the jacket top in place, he wore a well worn black belt. The boy could see that the belt was tied in the traditional way and at the end of the belt was four distinctive red tags, denoting that this instructor was a fourth dan black belt. This was indeed a high grade and the boy felt inwardly excited.

After about ten minutes, the Sensei beckoned him over to the side of the tatami (mat area). The boy approached and made a small bow to the Sensei. The Sensei politely returned the bow and with a smile on his face asked, "How can I help you?" "Sensei" the boy said "with your permission I would like to join your class and become one of your students". The smile had disappeared from the Sensei's face and he replied, "I'm afraid that this is not possible" The boy felt extremely disappointed but did not show that to the Sensei. The boy gave a small bow to the Sensei and said, Thank for your time Sensei" he turned and was about to walk away when the sensei said, "What is your name?" "James" the boy replied. "Well James", the Sensei said, "come back in a weeks time and we will see if this class is still for adults only, the numbers have dwindled on this class and I am trying to launch a new class that will be for all ages". The boy smiled and said "I will Sensei". He returned each week for the next couple of months until finally the class has changed from an adult education class to a general all comers Ju-Jutsu class and that is how over four decades ago, I, the boy then started my long career in Ju-Jutsu.

I often look back on those days and realise that I was really uninformed about what I was actually getting into; Ju-Jutsu was for me just another martial art. I had no idea just how involved this fantastic art was or how many different style there are in this art. On reflection I also believe that this is true of anyone who is just starting out in the martial arts.

We all find a club, (Dojo) that is convenient to where we live and that suits our pockets, but do we know anything about the art itself?

Well, I always have the excuse that over four decades ago there was no internet and any research would have been done by going to the local library and believe me, martial arts books were extremely limited back then . The big city libraries would have probably had a better selection of books but back then all I wanted to do was a learn Ju-Jutsu and, to be quite honest, I thought Ju-Jutsu was the same the world over............. How wrong I was!

So what is Ju-Jutsu and where did it come from?

Well to answer that question we must look back to its origins. Ju-jutsu (柔術) literally means the "art or science of softness" or literally translates to "the art of pliance". Wow! That makes it sound like some kind of gentle, almost placid art but primarily Ju-Jutsu was the art of the Samurai Warrior of feudal Japan! There was nothing gentle or placid about these fierce warriors.

Samurai (侍) was a term for the military nobility of pre-industrial Japan. The word "samurai" is derived from the archaic Japanese verb "samorau," changed to "saburau," meaning "to serve"; thus, a "samurai" is a servant, i.e. the servant of a lord.

It is believed by some historians that warriors and foot-soldiers in the "6th century" may have formed a proto-samurai; these warriors were highly skilled with various weapons and if caught in close quarter battle they were also proficient at grappling. This grappling took the form of striking (kicking and punching), throwing (body throws, joint-lock throws, unbalance throws), restraining (pinning, strangulating, grappling, wrestling). Defensive tactics included blocking, evading, off-balancing, blending and escaping. All of these methods combined to form the first rudimentary Ju-Jutsu.

In battle field conditions and other instances where the opponent was wearing amour, it was recognized that it was extremely difficult to dispatch a person or persons with striking techniques alone. So the most efficient methods for neutralizing an enemy took the form of powerful joint locking and breaking techniques, certain throwing techniques and deadly strangulation/choking techniques.

It must be understood that at this period of time and for many years to follow the "grappling techniques" of the Samurai Warriors were always secondary to their weaponry skills. It was not until the Muromachi period (1333-1573) that unarmed combat known as Nihon Koryu Ju-Jutsu (Japanese old style Ju-Jutsu) became known. With this in mind we must recognize that from the sixth century up to the Muromachi period, the techniques used and developed by the Samurai, are the foundation techniques that we build our Ju-Jutsu arts upon today.

So how long has "grappling" been around? Well man has been fighting since he first evolved on this planet and right from day one he has been developing his grappling skills. Some of the earliest records are found in a Chinese text written in the sixth century BCE that rank "wrestling" as a military skill on par with archery and chariot racing. What can be concluded from this is that grappling was not exclusive to Japan and that many civilisations had developed forms of unarmed fighting skills that go back hundreds of years, well before the warriors known as samurai.

A question must pop into your head, who founded Ju-Jutsu? The answer is no one individual founded Ju-Jutsu. It was developed as a necessity out of endless internal wars in feudal Japan. It was forged by the death and suffering of those who stood in its way and invented by long forgotten unsung heroes who lived and died using its techniques and principles.

One of the first recorded Ju Jutsu schools was founded by Prince Hisamori Takeuchi of Japan in 1532 and is named; Hinoshita Toride Kaizan Takenouchi-ryū (日下 捕手 開山 竹内流) although it is famous for its ju-jutsu. Takenouchi Ryū is actually a complete system of martial arts including armed grappling (*yoroi kumiuchi*), staff (*bōjutsu*), sword (*kenjutsu*), sword drawing (*iaijutsu*), glaive (*naginatajutsu*), iron fan (*tessenjutsu*), restraining rope (*hojōjutsu*), and resuscitation techniques (*sakkatsuhō*).

Ten years after that the Yōshin-ryū (楊心流?) was founded in 1632, by physician, Akiyama Shirōbei Yoshitoki in Nagasaki

Over the next few decades other famous (Ryu's) schools were also founded, such as;

- Sekiguchi-ryū (関口流?), or Sekiguchi Shinshin-ryū (関口新心流?), founded in 1640, notable for its Kenjutsu, Iaijutsu and Jujutsu.

- Sōsuishi-ryū (双水執流?) is a traditional Japanese martial art founded in 1650, a bujutsu school that focuses on Kumi Uchi (jujutsu) and Koshi no Mawari (iaijutsu and kenjutsu).

- And the famous Hontai Yōshin-ryū (本體楊心流?) is a traditional (*koryū*) school of Japanese martial arts founded 1660, by Takagi Shigetoshi. All of the above mentioned ryu (schools) are still in existence today and have branches throughout the world.

From it origins in Japan, the spread of Ju-Jutsu throughout the world is one that is has taken many years and has had many pioneers that have there own unique tale to tell. Regretfully some of these Ju-Jutsu pioneers tales have been lost through time and lack of documentation but a few are well documented and to give you the reader some idea of this historical Ju-Jutsu journey and the type of people who took it, I would like to take you on a small global trip that hopefully gives a small insight into how Ju-Jutsu came to various countries.

To portray this to you correctly, I will from time to time fill in the whys and wherefores of ancient Japanese culture and some of the philosophies behind the ideals of some the people I am about to mention.

My tale starts in England with a British railway engineer who had worked in Japan by the name of Edward William Barton-Wright; and he is credited as being the person to bring the art of Ju-Jutsu to England.

Edward William Barton-Wright had trained in Japan under various Ju-Jutsu styles and also Judo, on his return to England he started a "New Art of Self Defence", this was in March 1899. He had an article published Pearson's Magazine that summed up the new arts concepts as:

a) To disturb the equilibrium of your assailant.

b) To surprise him before he has time to regain his balance and use his strength.

c) If necessary to subject the joints of any parts of his body, whether neck, shoulder, elbow, wrist, back, knee, ankle, etc. to strains that they are anatomically and mechanically unable to resist.

This is the basis of Ju-Jutsu; he combined the skills that he had learned in Japan with boxing, savate and French stick fighting and named his system Bartitsu. This is not a joke! This was the real name and not something out of the cartoon "The Simpsons". Joking apart, Barton Wright was an influential man and through his liaisons with various Japanese masters, he arrange for two Japanese instructors to come to England and to instruct at his school called the Bartitsu Academy of Arms and Phyical Culture, also known as the Bartitsu Club. Those instructors were Yukio Tani and Sadakazu Uyenishi.

By 1903 the Bartitsu Academy of Arms and Physical Culture had closed its doors due to lack of interest, poor management and high fees and the two Japanese instructors Yukio Tani and Sadakazu Uyenishi carried on to inspire many, many others to take up Ju-Jutsu.

This tale has a sad ending to it. Edward William Barton-Wright in his day was an entrepreneur, good athlete and pioneer who had great insight into martial arts, but he died in 1951 at the age of 90 with no money and is alleged to have been buried in an unmarked pauper's grave.

Another amazing historical Englishman that has had an enormous impact on Ju-Jutsu and fighting arts was William Ewart Fairbairn. He was born February 28, 1885 in Rickmansworth, Herts, England (1885-1960). Fairbairn served with the British Royal Marine Light Infantry starting in 1901. During his tour of duty he successfully competed in and developed new methods for bayonet fighting and was classed by his equals and peers as a "rather good man in a dust-up".

After joining the Shanghai Municipal Police in 1907, he studied jujutsu under Professor Okada, a Japanese Jujutsu expert and bonesetter teaching in Shanghai, and at one time, personal instructor to the Emperor of Japan. He then studied Chinese martial arts under the direction of Tsai Ching Tung, who at one time was employed at the Imperial Palace, Peking, as an Instructor to the Retainers of the late Dowager Empress.

From his vast experiences Fairbairn developed his own fighting system named Defendu and taught it to members of the Shanghai Police force in order to reduce officer fatalities.

Defendu systems are still taught today by close quarter combat specialists around the world. They do not class Defendu as a martial art but as a Close Quarter Combat method of survival.

During WWII Fairbairn was recruited by the British Secret Service as an Army officer; he trained UK, US and Canadian Commando forces, along with Ranger candidates in close-combat, pistol-shooting, and knife-fighting techniques.

Fairebairn's career was one of inspiration to many who have studied fighting systems and it is speculated in a television series 'Secrets of War' that he was the possible inspiration for Author Ian Fleming's fictional MI-6 secret agent, James Bond.

4

Now you may be thinking that it is only swash buckling men and Japanese Ju-Jutsu masters that have had an influence on British Ju-Jutsu, but I have to tell you that certain Women were also showing the British public that they were no push over when it came to learning Ju-Jutsu and defending themselves.

Emily Diana Watts began learning Jujutsu in 1903 at Golden Square in Soho London under the instructorship of Sadakazu Uyenishi. Three years later, Emily Watts was running her own Ju-Jutsu club at Prince's Skating Rink in Knightsbridge. She must have been the first female to open a Ju-Jutsu club in Britain.

In 1906, Emily's very own Ju-Jutsu book, *The Fine Art of Jujitsu* was published with an impressive introduction by the Duchess of Bedford. This too must have been a first in Britain.

Although Emily Watts was one of the early pioneers for British woman in martial artists, she certainly wasn't the first, although she was probably one of the most affluent.

A well known suffragette of that period was Edith Garrud. Edith was the wife of William Gurrud and they were both students of Uyenishi. When Uyenishi left Britain in 1908 William Gurrud assumed the responsibility of teaching the men while his wife, Edith, taught the women and children. For anyone to be given the responsibility of teaching in the Uyenishi Dojo, it was indeed a great honour and for Edith to be acknowledge as a female Ju-Jutsu instructor was typical of the Japanese attitude towards women. In Japanese ancient culture women where recognised as warriors and even Samurai. History reflects the relatively strong position women held in samurai society at the time. Laws governing the shogun's court in the early 13th century allowed women equal rights of inheritance with brothers and the right to bequeath property. Samurai and bushi wives had high status in the household. They controlled household expenditure, managed servants, and were called upon to defend the home in times of war.

What amazes me is the popularity of women participating in Ju-Jutsu back then when you have to remember that British Women did not have a vote, and in most cases women were treated as second class citizens. Note; the vote was eventually granted to some women in 1918 and to all in 1928.

Europe

I can only speculate on this, but it is logical that certain European countries would have had insight into Ju-Jutsu systems well before England. The Dutch and Portuguese were trading with Japan in the 16th Century; this trading must have given them exposure to Japanese culture and the martial arts. Unfortunately no records are available to prove or disprove this.

I do know for certain that Ju-Jutsu was definitely in Europe about the same time as it entered into England. This is thanks to the spread of popularity in the early development of Jigoro Kano's Judo.

Jigoro Kano is the person who founded Judo, but back then it was not called Judo it, was called *Jiu Jitsu!* And also spelt this way.

Jiudo as it was spelt then, was the term that was selected by Professor Kano to better describe his Jiu Jitsu system. In 1905 a book was published, titled, *The Complete Kano's Jiu Jitsu.* The significance of this book and Kano's system was far reaching as it had been adopted in Japan as the official jiu-jitsu of the government in the army, navy, and police departments. It was the opinion of the Kano system practitioners that the older and "greatly inferior systems" had begun to drop into disuse. The newer generation in Japan was devoting its attention entirely to the Kano methods.

So what was so different in this new Jiudo Jiu Jitsu system? The following are the major points Kano set out in the modernizing of jiu jitsu (Ju-Jutsu).

1. Kano wanted Ju-Jutsu recognised as a modern sport, so this meant the exclusion of techniques with a "murderous intent". Kano still utilised the dangerous techniques of jujitsu but they were only taught on the principle of defence and not offence.

2. Kano's Judo had to be strong and possess substantial political power to convince the more combative jujitsu styles to officially unite as Judo. Kano wanted not just Japan but the world to know that Judo was a gentleman's art as he was an educator of high moral-social status,

 it played an important role in the path to success.

3. While omitting dangerous techniques, judo maintained the appeal of maintaining combat techniques to defeat opponents.

4. Kano insisted that all Judo students benefit both physically and ethically from the practice of this art.

As early as 1901, Ju-Jutsu Converts to the Kano methods had travelled to various European countries and were performing in circuses, "taking on all comers" and amazing audiences with their skill. The prize to defeat one of these "wrestlers" was £1 for lasting each minute or £50 for winning! This was an absolute fortune then, so you can imagine that there was never a shortage of challengers.

Even the European royalty were taken with this new method of combating. In 1901 German Kaizer Wihelm II (born *Prince Frederick William Albert Victor of Prussia*) was so impressed he invited two Japanese instructors to teach in the military school at Keil, and later Agitaro. One of whom taught jujutsu at the Berlin Military Academy.

Scandinavia

February 10, 1904–September 5, 1905 was the start and finish of the Japan- Russian war. Sweden was at that time an archenemy of Russia, and with the Russians defeated, the bonds between Sweden and Japan were strong. This bond was to manifest itself in the interest for jujutsu.

The first Swede familiar with jujutsu, was probably Viking Cronholm (1874-1961) a Swedish physiotherapist, boxer and elite-sportsman. Cronholm went to South Africa in 1904. It was there that he learned Ju Jutsu from an English officer. When he returned to Sweden he immediately introduced Ju-jutsu to his old boxing friends. The first official Ju-Jutsu exhibition given by Cronholm followed by a course in self-defence was held in January 1908. Cronholm spend most of his life in training the police, army and others in self defence.

Cronholm´s well known book "Jiu-jitsu Tricks" from 1908 has been published in more than 30 editions and was on sale into the 1990s. This would make it one of the most popular sports-books in Sweden. Many tens of thousands of Swedes had also been instructed in Ju-Jutsu by Viking Cronholm. He was even a pioneer in the teaching of Ju-Jutsu to women; his wife Ester participated in demonstrations in the early part of the century, and was very adept at Ju-Jutsu.

During the first half of the 20th century, there were several persons that gave courses in self-defence. The courses varied in quality. These persons were: Alex Weimark (1895-1953), Thorild Lundin (1909-1995), Artur Lidberg (1894-1968), Ernst Wessman (1900-1964), Einar Thunander (1893-1982) amongst others. They didn't teach jujutsu as a sport, only as self-defence.

U.S.A.

President Ulysses Grant was reported as the first American to observe a Jujitsu demonstration by Jigoro Kano, who was nineteen years old at the time, during a visit to Japan in 1879.

One of the earliest pioneers of Ju-Jitsu in the USA was President Theodore Roosevelt. He was a passionate enthusiast of this art and one of his first instructors was J. O'Brien. J. O'Brien learned JU-Jutsu while living in Nagasaki Japan and upon his return he was fortunate to have as one of his first students, the President of the United States of America.

Theodore (Teddy) Roosevelt was so enthusiastic that he also engaged the services of a Japanese instructor Yoshiaki Yamashita. Yoshiaki Yamashita was the first to be dispatched from Japan to demonstrate the Kano Ju-Jutsu/judo system.

Both J. O'Brien and Yoshiaki Yamashita gave lessons to the President in the White House basement. However Theodore (Teddy) Roosevelt would often give practical demonstrations to friends and White House Staff in other parts of the White House. In the words of President Theodore Roosevelt; "Every American athlete ought to understand the Japanese system thoroughly. You know, I practically introduced Ju-Jutsu to the Americans".

Yoshiaki Yamashita carried on to do great things to expand the the Kano Ju-Jutsu/judo system and even taught "nagewaza" (throwing) techniques of to the wives of Senators Lee and Wadsworth. J. O'Brien was particularly active in inspiring the USA police departments to take up a Ju Jutsu program. By 1930 the States Penitentiaries, Seattle PD, New Jersey State Police, Jackson (Michigan) all had jujutsu programs in place.

Hawaii

Henry Seishiro Okazaki was born in Japan in 1890 and today he is commonly considered to be the Father of American Jujitsu. Okazaki went to Hawaii when he was 17 years old and studied several different schools of Ju Jutsu as well as Okinawan Karate, Chinese Kung-Fu, Hawaiian Lua, Fillipino Knife fighting, American Boxing, and wrestling.

A heavy weight boxer by the name of Carl "K.O" Morris unwittingly put Okazaki on the Ju-Jutsu map when he accepted a Ju-Jutsu versus boxing match in September 1922. Morris had already beaten several Japanese martial arts experts in similar bouts prior to this match and Okazaki decided to restore Japanese honour by taking on this challenge. The fight was no push over for Okazaki who had his nose broken in the first round. In the second round Okazaki caught Morris's arm and applied a reverse arm lock and that ended the bout with Morris put down for the count. In 1924, he toured Japan, making an exhaustive study of several other styles of Jujitsu and also earned a third degree black belt in Kokodan Judo. He also made a special study of restorative massage, because he recognized the virtue of reversing the effects of deadly or disabling arts by restoration and treatment.

By 1930 Okazaki had moved from Hilo to Honolulu, and there he began teaching what he now called "Danzan Ryu" jujutsu. Henry Seishiro Okazaki died in 1951 however he left a fantastic legacy "Danzan Ryu" jujutsu. Many famous American Ju-Jutsu martial artists have studied this system and they themselves have gone on to write there own piece of Ju-Jutsu history and also to become living Ju-Jutsu legends.

Brazil

George Gracie left the shores of Scotland in 1801 and moved to the state of Para in north eastern Brazil; he settled in this area with his family for many years. Little did he know that this move would start a revolutionary turn in Ju-Jutsu nearly two hundred years into the future.

As we have established, Kano's students travelled far and wide and in 1914, Mitsuyo Maeda who had visited numerous other countries as an envoy for the Japanese government, arrived with the purpose of helping establish a colony in Brazil and also the help the colony prosper.

Whilst in Brazil Maeda met up with a descendent of George Gracie, Gastao Gracie who was now a very influential business man. Gastao Gracie son Carlos began to study under Maeda and became a great exponent of the art. It was with his brother Helio that they set what is known today and all over the martial world as Gracie Jiu-Jitsu or Brazilian Jiu-Jitsu. This system took the martial arts fighting world by storm with contests called the Ultimate Fighting Challenge (U.F.C) that were first held in the U.S.A and now are televised around the world. When one looks at modern Gracie Jiu-Jitsu in the fighting arenas you can definitely see that this style is based on classic Kano Judo.

The Gracie organization is now headquartered in California, and has worldwide schools. Importantly, Brazilian Jiu-jitsu has influenced Mixed Martial Arts. Mixed Martial Arts are combinations of several styles. Brazilian Jiu-Jitsu provides the basis for most of the ground fighting in MMA.

Ju-Jutsu Judo???

I know by now that you may be totally confused as to what is Ju-Jutsu and what is Judo, well back in the 1900 and for quite a few years to follow they were one and the same. The Japanese government itself did not officially mandate until 1925 that the correct name for the martial art taught in the Japanese public schools should be "judo" rather than "jujutsu. The divide came further as Judo became more and more of a sport and was eventually allowed into the Olympic Games in 1964. By this time Judo was definitely Judo. What did happen though is through Judo's transitional years, a number of styles and schools of Ju-Jutsu were completely eroded away and or they changed styles to keep up with the modern judo.

New Zealand

While many countries have had famous masters and martial pioneer's influences the spread of Ju-Jutsu one tale needs to be told and that is of a women who may have pioneered Ju-Jutsu into New Zealand and possibly Australia, and that is Florence "Flossie" LeMar that was the stage name of Florence Gardiner.

It is believed that Florence was born either in New Zealand's South Island or in Australia circa 1885. She spent her youth in New Zealand and showed special skills in athletics, becoming both a champion swimmer and skater during her teen years where her first claim to fame lay in giving exhibitions of the obscure sport of barefoot skating.

By 1913 she had married Joe Gardiner, an immigrant from England. Joe worked as a professional wrestler and showman. Joe is believed to have coached Florence in the skills of jujutsu, which he may have learned while in England. The two then developed a theatrical performance in which Florence delivered a lecture on the benefits of jujitsu as a means of self defence and physical culture, especially for women and children, followed by a series of skits in which she demonstrated a variety of jujitsu techniques against Joe playing the role of a hooligan. The show was described as being "a refined Vaudeville novelty for all the family" and the act toured music halls and variety stages throughout Australasia. As they travelled from city to city the pair also offered Jujutsu classes to the general public.

In 1913 the couple wrote a book entitled *The Life and Adventures of Miss Florence LeMar, the World's Famous Ju-Jitsu Girl*. This must have been quite a revelation at its time. The first half of *Life and Adventures* illustrates and explains a selection of Jujutsu techniques and in the second half there follows a selection of short chapters in which Flossie, the Worlds Famous Jiujitsu Girl, recounts a series of international adventures in which her Jujutsu skills were tested to the utmost. She is pitted against a range of adversaries including a villainous New Orleans gambler armed with a vial of acid, and an "escaped lunatic" in London who believes that he is a bear!

Harry Baldock is another New Zealand martial arts pioneer. He was borne in 1906 in Great Britain and emigrated with his family at the age of five. Harry's legacy began with his entry into Ju-Jutsu, Self defence and unarmed combat. He first began training in Christchurch in 1921 at the age of fifteen and then moved to Dunedin in 1929. Harry also had a distinguished army career and rose to the rank of Sgt Major, and it was in the army that Harry developed his military unarmed combat skills.

Harry Baldock was not just involved in martial arts, he was also a pioneer of body building, fitness and wrestling, his mentor for this was the legendry former New Zealand and Australian champion Jack Clarke.

In 1930 he opened up his own full time facility, the Baldocks Institute in Dudedin New Zealand. This institute is still open today and is now run by one of Harry's loyal students and friends, Tank Todd. Tank still teaches the Baldocks system along with his own legendry military unarmed combat system.

Jiu-Jutsu? Ju-Jitsu? Ju-Jutsu?

Before I go any further, I think I need to explain the different spelling of the name Ju-Jutsu."Jiu-Jitsu" was also the original spelling of the art in the West and that is why this style retains the original (although technically incorrect) spelling. Other common spellings are Jujitsu, Ju-Jitsu, Ju jitsu and Ju-Jutsu – the last being correct in accordance with modern Romanization.

"Ju-Jutsu" was not the name used originally, as it had several other names; (体術 **taijutsu**), (組討 or 組打 **kumiuchi**), (和術 **wajutsu**), (捕手 **torite**), (子具足腰之周 **kogusoku koshi no mawari**) and (柔道 **jūdō**). I know all Judo people out there are now jumping up and down but if you do your research this name was associated with Ju-Jutsu as early as 1724, almost two centuries before Kano Jigoro founded the modern art of judo!

It was not until the Edo period (1603-1868) that Ju-Jutsu became a generic term used to describe this wide range of techniques. This period is considered the "Golden Age" of Ju-Jutsu, when the major schools flourished and techniques were brought to its highest level.

In the Edo period Ju-Jutsu Ryu's (schools) started take on a look that is recognizable to the practitioners of Nihon jujutsu as seen today. The techniques were being developed and implemented to deal with opponents not wearing traditional armour nor in a battlefield environment. Most systems of Edo Ju-Jutsu included extensive use of atemi waza (vital area striking technique), which would be of no use against an armoured opponent on a battlefield! They would, however, be quite valuable in confronting an enemy or attacker during peacetime dressed in normal street clothes.

Another important development occurred towards the end of the Tokugawa period (1868) and that was the opening of Gendai Ju-Jutsu schools. These are modern Ju-Jutsu schools and at that point of time it is estimated that more than **"2000 koryu and gendai schools (ryu) existed"**.

Authors Note: I must say that I can sit here and laugh at this number, even by today's standards that would have been a complete saturation of the martial arts market and it makes one wonder just how many students did they have in each school? And how long did each school last? If the numbers attending each school were poor then I would say that some schools opened and closed their doors pretty quickly. I would also speculate that for the first time in the history of Ju-Jutsu the traditional ryu's (schools) changed their policies and opened their doors to all comers and not just the elite Samurai and upper classes. Another bit of speculation on my behalf is, the open door policy would bring in hefty financial revenues and that would ensure the survival of the Ryu (school).

While a few hundred Koryu Ju-Jutsu schools (old style Ju-Jutsu) still exist, Gendai Ju-Jutsu schools (modern style Ju-Jutsu) make up the majority of the worlds population of Ju-Jutsu schools in existence today. Ju-Jutsu systems are today codified practices and traditions of training for combat. They may be studied for various reasons including combat skills, self-defense, weapon skills, fitness, sport, self-cultivation/meditation, mental discipline, character development and building self-confidence, or any combination of the above.

There is a great diversity and abundance of Ju-Jutsu schools but, broadly speaking, Ju-Jutsu arts share a common goal: to defeat a person or persons physically or to defend oneself from physical threat.

It is this diversity that makes Ju-Jutsu an art within arts. Ju-Jutsu is recognised as the mother art from which other arts have developed from. Over time, the art was adopted by various groups of people who took different aspects and developed them much further than before. Karate, with its kicks, punches and numerous strikes, Aikido, with its elegant throws and powerful joint locks and Judo its throws, grappling, groundwork, arm locks and

strangulations all have a fundamental descendancy from these ancient techniques.

What makes Ju-Jutsu even more unique is that today there are so many different styles and interpretations of the art that to try to catalogue them all we be a mammoth task. I myself have studied; Goshin Jutsu, Atemi Jutsu, Tai Jutsu and Kempo Ju-Jutsu and have gone on to develop my own style Eikokyu Ryu Tai Jutsu Ju-Jutsu. Even this small list is so different in character and substance that when viewed by an outsider they would look like completely different martial arts.

So what is the best style of Ju-Jutsu to study?

That question can only be answered by you as it all depends on what you personally want from Ju-Jutsu. Most clubs Sensei's will be happy to explain the ideology of their particular Ju-Jutsu system, but you need to sit down and make up a list of your own personal goals and requirements. If the club you visit fits your listed agenda, then that is the club for you, if however none or only one or two of your chosen criteria are fulfilled then keep trying other clubs until you find what you are looking for.

The last paragraph may sound a little ambiguous for someone who are just starting out in martial arts as you may not know what you want from a Ju-Jutsu style or club, so to help you I have compiled a "What do I want from a Ju-Jutsu Club" listing to help steer you in the right direction.

What do I want from a Ju-Jutsu Club listing? ☑ Or × the box's ☐

Location: Is the club in a good location for me to travel too, Yes ☐ No ☐ and from ☐ Is there car parking, Yes ☐ No☐. Buses, is the bus stop or bus station close? Yes ☐ No ☐

Convenience: Are the class times convenient with my schedule? Yes ☐ No ☐

First impression: Is the club friendly? Yes ☐ No ☐

Hygiene: Is the club nice and clean? Yes ☐ No ☐

Classes: What is the objective of the class? Self Defence ☐ Combat skills ☐ Sport ☐ Weapon skills ☐ Fitness ☐ Building self-confidence☐ Character development ☐ Anti bullying ☐ other ☐

Men, Women and Children: Are the classes suitable for Men ☐ Women ☐ Children ☐ Mixed Classes☐ Men only ☐ Women only ☐ Children only ☐

Equal opportunity policy: Does the club have an Equal opportunity policy? Yes☐ No ☐

Spectator: Can I watch a class before I start? Yes ☐ No☐. Will it cost me anything to watch? Yes ☐ No ☐

Safety equipment: Does the club have the necessary safety equipment; good quality mats (tatami) to train on et cetera? Yes ☐ No ☐

Uniform (Gi): Do I have to buy a uniform before I start? Yes ☐ No☐. If yes, how much will a uniform cost? Good price ☐ Expensive☐. Or can I try a class in jogging bottoms and a loose top? Yes ☐ No ☐

Note: If you want to buy a suit (Gi), buy one that is suitable for Ju-Jutsu. You can buy light polyester/ cotton suits that are cheap, but they will tear easily when pulled using the typical Ju-Jutsu technique. The best ones to buy are Judo suits for the young children and adults or tournament karate suits for adults. Both of these are very strong and will last you a long time.

You may also have to buy a pair of Zori (dojo slippers or flip flops) for walking around the outer areas of the dojo.

Ventilation: Some Ju-Jutsu classes are held in tiny, poorly light and claustrophobic rooms, so is the club, dojo well ventilated? Yes ☐ No ☐

Health and Safety: Does the club have a health and safety policy? Yes ☐ No ☐

Class structure: Are the classes structured properly? Introduction, Yes ☐ No ☐ Warm up, Yes ☐ No ☐ Break falls, Yes ☐ No ☐ Student's safety, Yes ☐ No ☐ Ju-Jutsu techniques broken down so you can understand and follow, Yes ☐ No ☐ Cool down, Yes ☐ No ☐

Etiquette: Does the club have good etiquette? Yes ☐ No ☐

Syllabus: Does the club have a structured grading syllabus? Yes ☐ No ☐

Price: Prices vary from club to club, so are the class fees what I can afford? Yes ☐ No ☐

Membership: How much does the club membership cost? ☐ Is this annual, Yes☐ No ☐ or life, Yes ☐ No ☐

Insurance: Does the membership include personal accident insurance, Yes ☐ No ☐ and public liability insurance? Yes ☐ No ☐

Senior Instructors Qualifications: What grade is the senior club instructor? 1st Dan ☐ 2nd Dan ☐ 3rd Dan ☐ 4thDan ☐ 5th Dan ☐ 6th Dan ☐ 7th Dan ☐ 8th Dan ☐ 9th Dan ☐ 10th Dan ☐

Senior Instructor: Does the senior instructor teach on all the classes? Yes ☐ No ☐

Other Instructors Qualifications: Some clubs delegate classes to other instructors, what grades do they hold? 1st Dan □ 2nd Dan □ 3rd Dan □ 4thDan □ 5th Dan □ 6th Dan □ 7th Dan □ 8th Dan □ 9th Dan □ 10th Dan □

Professional Indemnity Insurance: Do all the instructors have Professional Indemnity Insurance and how much cover do they have? 1 million £ or $ □ 2 million £ or $ □ 3 million £ or $ 4 million £ or $ □ 5 million £ or $ □ or more □ In the UK the average is £2 million for amateur instructors and £5 million for professional instructors.

Affiliation and Association membership: What association or federation is the club affiliated too?□

Licence: Will I be issued a licence from that association Yes□ No □ and how much will it cost? Fair price□ To expensive □

Gradings: How often does the club do gradings? Each month □ two months □ three months □ four months □ five months □ six months □ or more □ and how much do they cost? Fair price□ Too expensive □

Club Contact number: Does the club have a land line contact telephone number; Yes □ No □ Does the club have a mobile telephone number; Yes □ No □ Does the club have an email address; Yes □ No □

Web site: Does the club have a web site? Yes □ No □

This list is just a basic guide and has not covered the actual contents of a typical Ju-Jutsu class, in the next few chapters; I will break down some of the components that are typical on a Ju Jutsu class so that you the reader can get a better overview of what Ju-Jutsu is about.

Bowing: when entering and leaving the Dojo.

So let's start from the beginning, bowing. As a student (Deshi)or as an experienced martial artist it is customary and polite to do a standing bow called Ritsu Rei as you enter or leave the Dojo (martial arts training hall). While a bow is just a physical act it shows a sign of respect to the Dojo you are about to enter or leave. The student (Deshi) traditionally would also use the standing bow (Ritsu Rei) as a way of clearing his or her mind in readiness for what they are about to learn or on leaving what they have learned. Most modern dojo's of today have lost this basic, but to me, important piece of etiquette.

How to perform the bow (Ritsi Rei):

Stand at the entrance to the Dojo(martial arts training hall) and remove your shoes. Face the Tatami (mat area) or if you know where the KAMIZA area is (upper seat). Stand upright with your feet together, hands by your side. Bend from the waist and do a small bow. When you are about to leave the Dojo (martial arts training hall): Perform the bow again.

Authors note: The bows done on a martial arts class have no religious meanings; they are simply a sign of respect, just the same as a hand shake would be used in the western world.

Reishiki, etiquette.

Reishiki is the etiquette and mat manners that are practiced in some but not all Ju-Jutsu Dojo's. Some just utilise parts of this and other are extremely strict on good etiquette. I believe that good etiquette is essential, it is part of the art we are studying and with good etiquette comes discipline and that in turn keeps the classes safe.

One of the reasons that reishiki is not practiced properly today is that an instructor hires a room in a leisure centre, scout hut or school hall to teach Ju-Jutsu and as the room is all things to everyone who hires and uses, the instructor/students seems to think that etiquette does not matter. How wrong they are! A dojo is a dojo no matter where it is whether it be a purpose built facility or your garage. Now that I have had my little rant, let's get back to reishiki.

To help you understand Reishiki and the rules of the Dojo at little better. I have includes a typical list of Dojo rules that are relevant to today's society.

The following rules and etiquette are to be observed at all times.

1. All members and none members will remove their shoes before entering the dojo.

2. No sweets, crisps, gum, food or beverages of any kind will be allowed on the Dojo.

3. By Law the Building has a no smoking policy. No smoking in the dojo or Building at any time by students or spectators.

4. No profanity or abusive language will be allowed in the dojo.

3. All members will bow entering and leaving the Dojo.

4. All members will bow to Sensei/Soke at the start and finish of each class.

5. All members will bow when coming onto and leaving the dojo Tatami (mat area). If a higher grade then yourself is on the Tatami, then stand on the side, raise your hand up to attract his/her attention and enter the tatami with a bow to that individual.

6. Personal cleanliness and hygiene are to be observed at all times. Your feet should be clean and odour free. Bring a towel with you so that you control your own perspiration. It is unhygienic and inconsiderate to sweat on other students!

7. Keep your fingernails and toenails short at all times.

8. Keep your uniform (gi) neat and clean at all times.

9. Do not wear rings, jewellery or any other metal ornaments in the Dojo when training

10. Do not leave personal belongings in the dojo changing areas.

11. Turn your mobile phone off when you enter the dojo.

12. Do not come to class while intoxicated. Do not consume any alcohol before a class or practice.

13. Do not run in the dojo.

14. Help students below your rank with knowledge.

15. Refrain from misusing your martial arts knowledge.

16. Do not show anyone who is not a club member any martial arts techniques and do not demonstrate in public.

17. Stay out of fights unless impossible to avoid. Report all fights to Sensei/Soke within 24 hours.

18. Do not criticize other members at anytime or other martial arts practioners.

19. Be on time for class, or inform the Sensei that you will be late.

20. The instructor is to be called Sensei/Soke at all times while in the dojo.

21. Signs and periodic postings are to be observed at all times.

22. Strive to promote the true spirit of martial arts by the development of:

    a) Respect (Courtesy to others)

    b) Character (Mental development)

    c) Humility (Never lose sight of your shortcomings)

    d) Health (Physical development)

    e) Skill (Proficiency in the arts you learn.)

Martial arts belts (obi) Kyū (級) & Mon Grade System.

The martial arts belt (obi) system started in 1880 under the Kano judo system, and at that point of time only two belts were used, the white and black. In the 1900s, the judo gi (Suit) was introduced and at around the same time the belt (obi) system expanded with a range of coloured belts that would denote the Judokas rank and competence. This belt system was then adopted by other Japanese martial arts.

In today's martial arts classes, a novice is someone who has not yet earned a belt (obi). Some older clubs start the novice with a red belt. In certain clubs, it is acceptable to wear a white belt with a red tag; the tag indicates that you are a novice; you then take the tag off when you earn your white belt.

As you train and become more proficient, you will be expected to take a grading. It is reasonable for grading to take place once every four months, some clubs extend this time and others trim it down. Gradings are also dependant on the amount of time you personally put in, if you only train once in a blue moon, don't expect to many gradings!

A grading is a way of assessing your progress, if you pass, you move to the next coloured belt. Most clubs will have a syllabus that specifies exactly what is required for each coloured belt. These syllabuses can vary greatly depending on the style and standard of the club; they can also change depending on if you are an adult or a child.

To give you a rough idea of what the belt colour system can be, you start by earning your white belt, then yellow, orange, green, blue, brown and then black. Different clubs and styles have added more colours to this, it is not unusual to see, purple or brown belts with white centre stripes.

The colour belt system is named, Kyu (級) grades. (Kyu (級) is pronounced 'Q' 'cue').

Kyu-level practitioners are often called *mudansha* (無段者), "ones without dan" or black belt.

The older Kyu (級) grade system starts at;

> 6th Kyu, white belt (the lowest kyu grade). The colour white signifies innocence.

> 5th Kyu, yellow belt. The colour yellow signifies the earth. The student begins to create a firm foundation in art, just as a seed begins to expand its root system deep in the earth as it begins to grow.

> 4th Kyu, orange belt. The colour orange signifies the changes of autumn, as the student's mind and body begin to develop and grow as a result of the new Ju-Jutsu experience.

> 3rd Kyu, green belt. The colour green represents growth, like that of the green plant as it sprouts out of the ground. The student has built a firm foundation and now begins to grow in the art

> 2nd Kyu blue belt. The colour blue represents the sky. Reminding the student to reach for the heavens and continue their martial arts journey.

1st Kyu, brown belt (the highest kyu grade). The colour brown represents the ripening or maturing process as that of the advanced student whose techniques are beginning to mature.

The colour black is the opposite of white and signifies maturity and dignity.

Please note: New Ju-Jutsu systems can start as low as 12th or 10th Kyu (級).

Junior grades can also be known as, Mon grades (translated as Gate in English). The maximum age of a junior is normally 16 years old.

The mon grade system has the same coloured belts as the kyu grade system, but adds coloured tags at each grade level to assist and encourage the junior through the grading process.

For example; a junior who is already a white belt and is taking the next grade level, yellow belt. He or she shows during the grading that they can only do certain movements within the set grade criteria. Instead of failing this junior, he or she is awarded one or two yellow tags towards the next yellow belt. These tags are called mon grade, each junior colour grade is made up with three mon tags.

Black belt, Dan (段 dan) Grade, Yūdansha (有段者), "one with dan".

YŪDANSHA (有段者) simply means "The one that has level". (Some people call them "DAN holder" in English".)

A black belt denotes a high degree of competence in that art but, it does not mean that the holder is a master. It is not until 5th or 6th Dan that one becomes a master. Some systems have also introduced 4th dan as a master grade, it will not be long before this drops to 3rd Dan!

The black belts are broken down into Dan grades, they are as follows;

Many Martial Arts use between one and ten dan ranks:

shodan (初段: しょだん): first degree black belt. (1st Dan, Being the lowest dan grade)

nidan (二段: にだん): second degree black belt

sandan (三段: さんだん): third degree black belt

yodan (四段: よだん): fourth degree black belt

godan (五段: ごだん): fifth degree black belt

rokudan (六段: ろくだん): sixth degree black belt

nanadan (七段: ななだん): seventh degree black belt (also, *shichidan*)

hachidan (八段: はちだん): eighth degree black belt

kudan (九段: く だ ん): ninth degree black belt

jūdan (十段: じ ゅ う だ ん): tenth degree black belt. (10th Dan, Being the highest dan grade)

Junior Black Belts.

Traditionally in Japan, the minimum age for black belt was 16 years of age. The reason was simple. A boy was not considered a man until he turned 16. The term Shodan, does not mean 1st dan or degree black belt. The word shodan is broken down into two words, Sho means 1st, dan means man. The Japanese felt that one must be mature enough to be a black belt.

In lots of countries around the world this policy had been adopted, however to get around the youth issue, a child can be graded as a junior black belt. This can give the child black belt recognition up to the age of sixteen. Once the teenager reaches sixteen, they can then move onto the senior dan grade scale.

Entering the Tatami (mats)

When you have entered the (Dojo) club, you may have to get changed into your Gi (suit) or suitable attire for training in. Once this is done this you will be ready to go onto the (Tatami) mats, but before you can do this another bow is in order , this time you will have to stand just off the mat area and then do a standing bow (Ritsu Rei). As before you will have to face the KAMIZA, so where is the KAMIZA area? The KAMIZA is the highest point of honour in a Dojo. It is the upper seat or seat of honour in which proper reishiki is reserved for the highest dan holders. In traditional Dojo's you can see this area straight away, as it will have a photo of the chief instructor or arts founder hung on the wall. It is speculated in days gone by that the Kamiza was the warmest and less draughty place in Dojo and that is where the head sensei would be, personally I like this suggestion.

To understand the layout of a Dojo and (Tatami) mat area is also good reishiki, so here is how it works:

Kamiza is the highest point or upper seat in the Dojo. This is where the Highest graded person would sit.

Joseki is the second most important area of a Dojo. If the sensei wishes, he may have any of the black belts (Yudansha) sit next to him on his left side. These would be in a grade order that descends from his left.

Shimoseki is the third area of importance in the Dojo. This is reserved for the lower dan grades and in modern times for the junior and intermediate black belts, youngsters up to the age of eighteen.

Shimoza is the lowest area of the Dojo. This is where all coloured belts line up in grade order from right to left; this will be opposite to the sensei. If you are novice, you would be at the bottom of the line. Don't worry, we all started at the bottom of the line but one day you will be at the top.

A typical class will start with the students standing in line on the tatami (mat area) in grade order (colour of belts and black belt ranks). At the order of one of the senior grades the word (seiza) is called and everyone will take a formal kneeling position. The command is then called "Sensei ni rei!" (Bow to the instructor).

How to do a Kneeling (seiza):

Take a small step forward with the right leg and place left knee on the mat; in an arc reverse the right foot back and kneel on the right knee. Sit down on your feet. The Big toes of left and right feet should overlap (it does not matter which toe is on top). Keep your back straight, head upright and shoulders relaxed. Rest left hand on left thigh with the hand open, fingers together. The right hand rests on the right thigh also with the hand open and fingers together. Both hands should point inwards. For anatomical reasons, men should have about a fist or two's width between their knees, women should have knees together.

Bowing in seiza:

Take the left hand from your left thigh and place it palm down on the Tatami (mat area) just in front of your left knee. Now take the right hand from your right thigh and place that palm down on the Tatami (mat area) just in front of your right knee. Bow slowly at the waist. Some schools bow very low and others make a polite bow so on this, just follow the instructors example. Once you have bowed, bring your hands back to your thighs. It is customary for the Students (Deshi) to remain seated until the black belts (Yudansha) stand up and then the students can also stand. Note: The etiquette of bowing at the start of a class is also repeated at the end of each class.

Zazen (seated meditation), Mokuso (focused meditation).

Some, but not all Ju-Jutsu schools practice some form of meditation whether it is Zazen (seated meditation), Mokuso (focused meditation). The idea of the meditation is to clear your mind. This is normally done just after the seiza (bow). To do this, start by inhaling in through your nose and let the breath go deep into the hara (the centre of gravity in the belly), then exhale out slowly through your mouth. As you breathe have your eyelids half-lowered, the eyes being neither fully open nor tightly shut, this way, you are not distracted by outside objects but at the same time it keeps you awake! So don't nod off. Mentally you should try to think of nothing, the mind become clear and ready to take in what you are about to learn.

Warming up and exercise

The next and very important part of the class is the warm up. The term "warm up" is a generalisation on martial arts classes for a whole range of exercises. Each club Sensei has their own format for this, but the prime objective is always the same and that is to; increase the level of physical fitness and overall health of each student. To put this in fighting terms, you have to be fit to fight.

Another way of looking at the warm up is; you are preparing the body for the exertion that is to follow. The body's temperature is raised and the heart rate is increased, which in turn raises the temperature of the muscles. In doing this, the fluid that is between joints is circulated, thus decreasing the chance of the ends of the bones grinding against one another, your muscles are primed for use and this will minimise pulls and strains. So by warming up properly you are protecting your own body.

The benefits of exercise are as follows: Taking regular exercise reduces the risk of heart disease and diabetes and all other horrible thing we can get from inactivity. Over a period of time it will increase your stamina. It can also help with weight control and also strengthening the body's immune system. Doing certain types of exercises will help shape your muscles, builds muscle strength, helps maintain healthy bone density, and joint mobility; and finally exercise promotes a physiological well-being.

The classes' physical exercise's can be broken down into the following;

Breathing exercises: This increases the oxygen taken into the body to where it is needed and expels carbon dioxide out of the body. Deep breathing exercises have a wondrous effect on you as it expels stale oxygen out of your of your body and replenishes it with fresh oxygen and this invigorates you both mentally and physically. You have to remember that breathing is good for you, without it you will die!

Stretching: There are hundreds of different ways of stretching out our muscles and a good stretch can simply be pleasurable. Most classes will have a good range of stretches that will help reduce muscle injury and they will also use stretching exercises that are designed to help lengthen the muscles, in order to increase muscle flexibility and/or joint range of motion.

Aerobic exercise: Aerobic means "with oxygen" This is the part of the class that gets you heart pumping and is good for strengthening the cardiovascular system. Exercises for this are numerous as aerobic exercises cover lots of body motion exercises. This is just a few examples: jogging on the stop, skipping, star jumps, squat thrusts and pad work.

General exercises: Such as sit ups or crunches are both aerobic exercise and anaerobic exercises depending on how many you do and what style of exercise you do them in. Sit ups or crunches are good for abdominal workout and if done properly these can help shape your abdominal muscles into that much desired six pack, but a healthy diet is also needed to shape them. Push ups are good for building upper body strength in the biceps, triceps and other localised muscles, but they can be difficult for women and young children. I always recommend that these be done "kneeling mode" for those who cannot manage a full press up.

Anaerobic exercise: Weight training and power lifting are anaerobic exercises. I have included this exercise range as sports Ju-Jutsu clubs and mixed martial arts classes encourage anaerobic exercise to build muscle mass. Muscles that are trained under anaerobic conditions develop biologically differently giving them greater performance in short duration-high intensity activities.

Resistance training: This type of exercise is one that I often use in my Dojo. I use the elastic resistance bands. They are quite cheap and extremely portable and fun to use. You can purchase them in different resistance strengths so everyone on the class can use them. Resistance training is a form of strength training in which each effort is performed against a specific opposing force generated by resistance (i.e. resistance to being pushed, squeezed, stretched or bent). Exercises are *isotonic* if a body part is moving against the force. Exercises are *isometric* if a body part is holding still against the force. Resistance exercise is used to develop the strength and size of skeletal muscles.

Once the warm up is over the class will normally go into Ukemi Waza(Break falling techniques).

U·ke·mi (受身). Waza (a Japanese word that means "technique").

Ju-Jutsu has numerous throws, sweeps and knock downs and that equates to you being thrown down on the tatami (mat area). If you are new to Ju-Jutsu, don't start panicking. Before you are thrown the club sensei (teacher) will teach you how to break your fall safely. In years gone by we would spend months just practicing break falls before we were allowed to do a throw! Unfortunately people of today are inpatient and want things instantly. Well this is one thing that is worth taking your time over, aslearning to break fall correctly will allow you to be thrown safely, without injury and you will enjoy your training. Skipping this or taking this lightly will only result in you being injured!

So how does the break fall work? To understand this you first of all need to understand about the tatami (mat).

Tatami (畳 *tatami*) (originally meaning "folded and piled") mats are a traditional Japanese flooring. Made of woven straw, and traditionally packed with rice straw (though nowadays sometimes with Styrofoam), tatami are made in individual mats of uniform size and shape, bordered by brocade or plain green cloth.

There are various rules concerning the number and layout of tatami mats; the mats must not be laid in a grid pattern, and in any layout there is never a point where the corners of three or four mats intersect as it is said to bring bad fortune, this is particularly true when they are laid in traditional Japanese homes.

Modern tatami are made up of high density chip foam, 1m wide x 2m long and 20mm to 40mm thick or 1m x 1m x 20mm to 40mm thick that can be bought in different densities which are covered in a tatami pattern PVC fabric. An alterative to this is the styrofoam jigsaw mat; each mat is 1m x 1m x 20mm to 40mm thickness with various densities. The density of the mat determines the mats structural resistance to impact.

Human equation:

Now that you have an idea of the construction of the mats, let's look at the next part of the breakfall equation, a human being. While the human body is reasonably resilient, if you throw that body onto a hard floor the body will suffer various injuries. The reason for this is the hard floor is a solid surface and our body is soft by comparison. When the body hits the floor, it is the body that absorbs the impact.

When you have a mat area (tatami) and we have already established that the tatami is made out of foam and you then throw a body onto this surface the foam will absorb some of the impact. The tatami (mat area), by its construction has broken some of the fall.

To understand a little bit more about falling, we must first go back to the "human being" and look at one of our most natural reactions. If you slipped over in the street and was about to fall on your back, what would you do? The answer is put your arms out to protect yourself and reduce the impact on the floor. How does this work? Well, by putting your arms out increases the amount of area that is about to hit the floor and that reduces of overall impact on the rest of the body.

A break fall works in exactly the same manner, as you are falling, you put an arm or arms out and that in effect reduces the overall impact as you hit the tatami (mat area).

The break fall (Ukemi) actually takes this a bit further because as you are about to land on the mat on your back you don't just put your arm out, you strike the mat with your hands open,(fingers apart) and forearms with some force. This now compresses the foam mat over the expanse of your arms width and breaks your fall. Once you strike the mat, you then have to pull your hands up away from the mat, thus allowing the mat to absorb the energy of the impact and stops the return of energy as the compressed foam mat starts to regains its initial shape.

The angle of you arms for break falling in relation to your body are optimised when they are held at about a forty five degree angle. This allows the arms to swing freely well past the upper torso and they hit the mar area (tatami) moments before the main part of the body makes contact with the mat. This reduces the imminent impact to a minimum.

Breathing and break falls.

When you practice your break falls it is important that you co-ordinate your breathing with the striking of the mat (tatami) with your arm or arms. This must be timed correctly - just as you are about to strike the mat (tatami), exhale sharply. This will stop you getting winded.

Breathing out when you hit the mat (tatami) also has another benefit! It can save you a little embarrassment! When we have air in our bodies, our bodies are like a balloon. If you do not breathe out when you hit the mat, you not only get winded but it can cause you to break wind! This is caused by the air in the lungs not being expelled and this can cause internal pressure on digestive tract, our digestive tract contains gas and this gas is then forced out through the rectum as the body impacts with the mat. Oh dear!

Mat density.

Mat (tatami) areas vary in density and thickness and this makes a big difference to the breakfall. If the mat is extremely soft then as you break fall you will hit the floor underneath as the foam has no resistance to your fall. This will result in pain and injury. The same is applied if the mat is too hard, the mat will not compress under the breakfall and again this will result in pain and injury. In most Dojo's (clubs) they have "Club Mats" that have the right balance of density and are comfortable to break fall on.

The thickness of a mat (tatami) will also make or break you! The ideal thickness is 40mm; the 20mm thick mats are not good for heavy break falls as you can often breakfall through the mat and hit the floor underneath!

Various forms of ukemi: Breakfalls

1. Yoko ukemi – a sideways fall. For a sideways break fall you use one arm to break your fall. The rule is; if you land on your right side you would use the right arm to break fall, landing on the left side, use the left arm to break fall with.

2. Ushiro ukemi – a backwards break fall. For this break fall you would use both arms. It is very important with this break fall to keep your head up as you land on the mat. The rule for this is; heads and mats don't mix!

3. Mae ukemi – front break fall. This break fall throws you face down, you break your fall with both hands (fingers open) and the forearms. There are two rules for this break fall; 1) never land on the palms of your hand with your arms straight! You will break your wrists doing this as all of your body weight is impacted through the wrists. 2) For safety turn your head to one side, it does not matter which side you turn your head. This will save you going face first into the mat!

Martial Art Rolls:

1. Zenpo Kaiten – forward roll. This movement is done when you are projected forward away from your training partner with your balance comptomised as opposed to break falling.

2. Ushiro Kaiten – backward roll. This movement is done when you are projected backwards away from your training partner as opposed to back break falling.

I have included both of these rolls into the Ukemi (break fall) range as both can be modified into a break falls. Zenpo Kaiten - forward rolls can be modified where you roll out of a throw (such as a small wrist turn) and then land in a side break fall. (Zenpo Kaiten - forward roll - Yoko ukemi - sideways fall).

Ushiro Kaiten – backward roll can be modified by doing a back break fall as you roll backwards, this help reduce the speed of the backwards roll. Ushiro Kaiten – backward roll - Ushiro ukemi- backward break fall.

Basics

When you first start a Ju-Jutsu class you can expect to start with the basics, in many cases this will mean learning about stances, how to block, punch and kick. Each of these are really important as these four items are the foundation of the art and all other techniques are built upon these.

Stances

What is a stance?

A stance in martial arts is a formal body posture that is often done in conjunction with other martial arts technique to help maximize the delivery of one or more techniques. For example; a forward stance (zenkutsu dachi) can be done with a rising block (age-uke) and then followed by a reverse punch (Gyaku-zuki)

Two of the most common stances are, forward stance and straddle stance.

Zenkutsu dachi: Forward or front stance. This stance is a common stance and is a major base stance whilst doing various blocking, punching and kicking techniques. It can also be used to assist in various locking methods.

To practice a basic forward stance, stand with your feet about your own shoulders width apart and then step directly forward about one and half shoulder widths with either the right or left leg. As you step forward bend from your front knee. You are now in a forward stance. Please remember this is a basic description, your club sensei (teacher) will show you the finer point of this stance.

kiba dachi: horse ridding stance / side stance / straddle stance. This stance has several names but they all refer to the same stance. I have personally found this stance extremely practical in Ju-Jutsu when utilized in numerous defense routines.

To practice a basic straddle stance, stand with your feet about your own shoulders width apart. Now pivot your right foot to your immediate right and step with your left foot forward so both the right and left feet are parallel and the bend equally from your knees, it is also important that you keep your back straight and upright. You are now in a straddle stance. If you reverse this process you will end up in a left straddle stance. To really understand how to do this correctly, seek advice from your sensei (teacher).

Other stances are; Fudo dachi: (rooted stance) hachiji dachi: (natural stance) kokutsu dachi: (back stance) neko ashi dachi: (cat stance). There are several other stances but they are utilised more in the Karate arts.

Fighting Stance

This is the stance that you will adopt most of the time when you are preparing to defend yourself; class wise or street wise. A fighting stance is more flexible than the other stances as you need to be able to move quickly from this stance into one of the more rigid stances when you are delivering a technique or techniques

To give you a basic idea of what a fighting stance is try the following. Bring one foot forward so that your feet are about your own shoulders width apart. Align your feet so that they are almost but not quite parallel and turn your front foot inward. The idea is to reduce visible target area to a minimum. Now bring your hands up to a guard position and you are in a basic fighting stance. I have only explained this basically, I would recommend that you seek advice from a sensei (teacher) who will explain the finer points of this stance.

Blocking Techniques (Uke-waza)

What is a blocking technique?

A blocking technique is a powerful range of techniques, utilising an arm or arms to stop an attacker from striking you with a blow to your person with there hands, fists, feet or knees or other parts of the their body.

A blocking technique can also stop an attacker's assault if they were armed with a weapon. Note: You should never block a weapon with your arms. Why? Because you will be seriously injured! Cautionary Note (I have to put this in!) In an armed attack, do not block the weapon with any part of your body, example; Head! Ouch! It is better to deflect or evade the weapon.

Blocking techniques are executed in conjunction with stances I have already listed and when done simultaneously, will help maximise the power of the blocking technique.

The following list is a range of blocking techniques that are quite common on Ju-Jutsu classes.

1. Jodan age-uke. Rising block. You would use this block for attacks coming downward towards your head. This type of attack would more than likely be a weapon attack.

2. Empi uke. Elbow block. This is a close quarter block and I do mean close quarter. Elbow blocks would deal with hooks and round house punches to the head or ribs.

3. Gedan baria. Downward sweeping block. Excellent for blocking low punches to the stomach, groin and certain low kicks.

4. Jodan Juji uke. Rising cross block. A rising cross block is a very powerful block. It is ideal for close quarter attack situations, for example; the attacker is armed with a cosh and he grabs a hold of your lapel with one hand and tries to strike you on the head with the weapon hand.

5. Gedan Juji uke. Downward cross block. Using this blocking technique correctly can save you from getting kicked in the groin! So it is well worth learning.

6. Shuto uke. Knife hand block. Aimed correctly this block is a "cut" above the others as it slices into the contact area, but this blocking technique also takes practice to

get it right.

7. Soto uke. Outside forearm block. This block is powerful block; it can deal effectively with some ferocious attacks to the head and the classic Saturday night special. Ok, just in case you don't know what a Saturday night special is, this a that big swinging punch thrown by drunks.

8. Sukui uke. Scooping block. Excellent range of blocking technique that teaches you how to evade, parry and trap front and side kicking techniques and can also be used against certain types of punches.

9. Ude uke. Inside forearm block. An extremely useful block for close quarter attacks to the side of the head or upper body.

Over the years that I have been studying martial arts, I have developed my own style of blocking techniques, these I call "block strikes". I utilise the same blocks that I have listed above but instead of just blocking an attack, the block strike is used to power though the attackers arm. I find this method very destructive and it also throws the attacker physically off balance.

Punches and hand techniques

In Ju-Jutsu the Japanese word for punch is Tsuki, however this is classed as a compound word that is virtually never used on its own. You would use this at the end of a range of words describing what kind of punch you are doing. For example Oi-Tsuki (lunge punch), but things get a little more complicated. Because it has been tagged on the end of a word its pronunciation and writing changes slightly; this is translated as zuki not tsuki.

Punches are complex techniques and have quite a few variations. To learn how to do a punch correctly you will need to be shown the correct way to close your hand in order to make a fist. And then you will need to be shown the technique of how to execute the punch. This should be done under the instruction of an experienced martial arts teacher.

The most common punches (zuki) in Ju-Jutsu are;

1. Gyaku-zuki (逆突き), reverse punch, a punch with the rear arm

2. Oi-zuki (追い突き), lunge punch, a punch with the lead arm

3. Age-zuki (上げ突き), rising punch, an upper cut.

4. Tate-zuki (立て突き), vertical fist punch into the middle of the chest (short-range)

5. Morote-zuki (双手突き), augmented punch using both hands

6. Mawashi-zuki (回し突き), hook punch also known as a round house punch.

Other important hand techniques. (Te waza)

Punches are only one way of using your hand or hands to strike with; the following list details other methods of hand striking techniques (Te waza).

1. HAITO UCHI "Ridge hand Strike". A good general strike, but it takes lots of practice. The strike is delivered with the thumb side of the hand.

2. KAISHO "Open hand." This refers to the type of blow which is delivered with the open palm. It can also be used to describe other hand blows in which the fist is not fully clenched.

3. TETTSUI UCHI "Hammer Fist Strike". An excellent all round hand technique that can "hammer" you into the ground.

4. NIHON NUKITE, "Two finger stabbing attack". Striking using this technique is restricted to vulnerable, softer areas only (Atemi)

5. NUKITE "Spear Hand". "Using four straight fingers". Striking using this technique is restricted to vulnerable areas only (Atemi)

6. OYAYUBI IPPON KEN "Thumb fist Knuckle". This is also a technique that is restricted to vulnerable areas only (Atemi)

7. SHUTO UKE "Knife-hand Block". Also SHUTO UCHI "Knife Hand Strike" This is a good hand technique, but you need to practice lots to be able to use it safely. This strike is delivered with the little finger side of the hand.

8. TEISHO UCHI "Palm Heel Strike". A good all round hand technique.

9. URAKEN UCHI "Back Knuckle Strike" or "Back Fist Strike".

To conclude, there are many types of hand techniques but you must be made aware of the dangers of making a mistake when using any of the above techniques. The human hand has twenty seven bones and it easy to break anyone of these, or even several bones in one go if you get it wrong! So get professional advice on how to do each hand technique and then practice until you perfect each individual hand technique. This has taken some martial arts masters a life time, so don't expect perfection after a couple of goes. Practice, practice and some more practice is the martial arts way.

Kicking Techniques (Geri-waza).

Despite what you may read or hear. Ju-Jutsu has quite a comprehensive range of kicking technique that equals any kicking art. What you have to remember is that all kicking techniques take lots of practise. I always recommend that if you are new to kicking techniques, start your practice low and slow, this way you will learn the techniques properly and you won't end up straining or pulling unnecessary leg muscles.

Each Ju-Jutsu club has its own method for teaching kicking techniques. Regardless of the method, try not to kick into thin air, you have no physical resistance to your kick and this can result in knee joint damage. It is much better and safer if you can kick into a proper kicking pad.

The following kicks are common on a Ju-Jutsu class.

1. Fumikomi geri: Stamping kick. For this kick, using the heel of the foot gives maximum impact power.

2. Hiza geri: Knee strike.

3. Mae geri: Front kick. This is a complex kick; it has several foot variations depending on the target area you are aiming for.

4. Mae-ashi mae geri: Front kick with front leg.

5. Mae tobi geri: Front flying kick.

6. Mawashi geri: Roundhouse kick.

7. Nidan tobi geri: Double jump kick.

8. Tobi geri: Jump kick.

9. Tobi ushiro mawashi geri: Jumping back roundhouse kick.

10. Ushiro geri: Back kick.

11. Ushiro kekomi: Back side thrust kick.

12. Ushiro mawashi geri: Reverse roundhouse kick.

13. Ushiro ura mawashi geri: Reverse back roundhouse kick.

14. Yoko geri keage: Side snap kick.

15. Yoko geri kekomi: Side thrust kick.

16. Yoko tobi geri: Jumping side kick.

Atemi (当て身)

Now that I have got the basics out of the way, I can now start to explain one of the fundamental elements that is can be used as a stunning stand alone art or as an intricate part of any Ju-Jutsu system.

The word Atemi (当て身) is a generalisation for the art of striking to vulnerable areas of the body.

Atemi Waza is the use of various designated blows and attacking techniques to vulnerable areas of the body that are used by numerous Ju-Jutsu systems.

Atemi Jutsu

Atemi Jutsu is the Ju-Jutsu art that includes all the normal elements that make up a Ju-Jutsu art but the radical difference is that it concentrates of strikes to key areas of the body. Those being: pressure points, nerve endings, numerous arteries running close to bone, internal organs, vulnerable joints like elbows and knees, fingers, wrists and sensitive regions such as the groin, eyes, ears and throat. To understand these points the student of Atemi needs to understand elementary anatomy of the human body. This can be learned over a period of time as to start with some of the atemi strikes are general basic strikes and the new student needs to also learn what parts of the body you use to strike with. The rule for this is simple, if you can hit with it, use it.

Kyusho Jitsu 急所術

Kyusho Jitsu, the striking of pressure points.

This art differs from Atemi Jutsu as it concentrates more on small targets on the body that are the pressure points of the body, as used in acupuncture. Each point has a different function and by interrupting this function with various extremely accurate strikes the proponent can cause the recipient extreme pain, unconsciousness or even death! Kyusho jitsu raised its profile in recent years by becoming somewhat controversial. Some of its experts have been scrutinised by the media and under test conditions they have not been able to live up to what they have personally claimed.

This does not make this a bad art to learn and study as one has to remember that the study of acupuncture has a rich and cultural history. And for those who have had acupuncture treatment, the relief from pain and suffering is indeed a god send. Even today our own medical scientists cannot explain how it works. It is interesting that some of the points used to injure and inflict pain on people in these arts are also used in the healing art of acupuncture and acupressure. What kills can cure and what can cure can kill!

History of Atemi.

Atemi's history can be traced back thousands of years ago to Asia and came under the

name Dim Mak (meaning death touch). With Chinese and Japanese cultural exchanges Dim Mak found its way into Japan under the name of Atemi. The Samurai of the battle field would have little use for this but as time progressed the Samurai integrated Atemi into there unarmed fighting systems.

It is said that the masters who developed this art toiled for a life time, attempting to perfect atemi. While they had a good knowledge of anatomy they also eagerly experimented on criminals and prisoners of war, testing the painful and sometimes lethal techniques! It is also speculated that atemi techniques were used to interrogate prisoners!

Irrespective of what the intention is, the basics of atemi traditionally are broken down into five elements. Through my own study of atemi, I found the five elements adequate but I felt they did not embrace comprehensively all of the aspects of atemi, so I have added three more elements, increasing this to eight elements in all. It should be noted that some of the elements cross over each other or have similarities; this is because they should all flow naturally together.

1, Accuracy:

As atemi waza is striking to key points of the body, the accuracy of that strike is vital. The atemi practitioner must hone his or her skills so that every strike lands perfectly on the designated target. For this the atemi practitioner must know instinctively the exact location of each target and have perfected all of the striking techniques.

2, Speed:

Any strike is more devastating when it is delivered with speed. This also applies to Atemi waza, with the more speed applied, the greater the impact and this results in a more successful delivery of the technique.

3, Maai (間合い), translating simply to "interval",

Maai Is a Japanese martial arts term referring to the space between two opponents in combat. As the attacker or attacker's out in the street has no specific size, the defendant has to gauge the distance of an effective blow or strike. This will vary greatly when you consider that some of the strikes will be with hand techniques in close proximity and other will be with foot techniques.

4, Route:

The route taken to deliver a successful atemi waza will vary from attacker to attacker. Each attacker will be attacking you in a different way. For example: the attacker has a knife and is trying to stab you with it, you may at first have to use evasive moments to avoid the knife, and then you may have to apply some form of lock to control the knife attacker's knife hand. After this you may have to use a throw in order to drive the attacker to floor. Finally you are now in a position to deliver the atemi or in some cases several atemi's to subdue the attacker.   The route taken has been but would be completely different if the attacker was in close proximity and trying to strangle you.

5, Angle:

Working on the assumption for every action there is a reaction; in delivering several atemi's (strikes) to the same person, the angle and position of their body will change as each strike lands. With experience, the atemi practitioner will be able to instantly adjust to the angle and find new targets.

6, Timing:

The delivery and timing of any blow in any martial art is important, and in atemi the decisive strike is maybe the only strike that is needed, so timing of that one strike is essential to victory. One has to understand that it is not easy to win with one strike and the opponent is not readily going to let this happen. Part of timing is also getting that person in a position

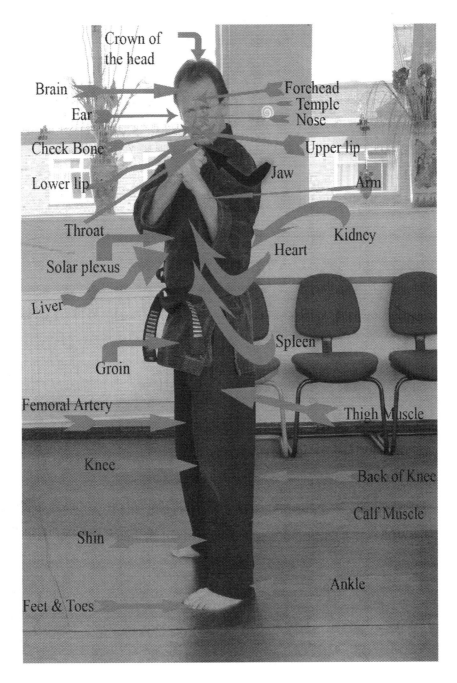

Illustration 1, a. Striking points front.

Striking Chart: back.

Illustration 2, a, shows the back of the body, again in a fighting stance, left leg forward and the various zones available to strike to.

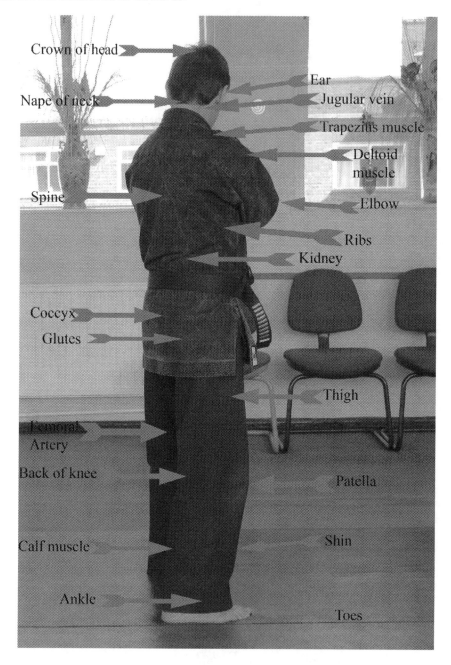

Crown of head

Ear
Jugular vein
Nape of neck
Trapezius muscle
Deltoid muscle
Spine
Elbow
Ribs
Kidney
Coccyx
Glutes

Thigh

Femoral Artery
Back of knee
Patella

Calf muscle
Shin

Ankle
Toes

Illustration 2, a.

The catalogue below is a typical "Atemi" list that names the part of the body and the type of strike that you can do to it. It is not a secret catalogue that I am revealing for the first time. Ancient lists and accurate atemi charts can now be found on lots of internet sites.

If you are unsure of any of the hand or foot techniques referred to in the list below, I have detailed these in my previous books, A breath of fresh air, Kempo karate, novice to intermediate and , A breath of fresh air, Kempo karate, intermediate to advanced by James Moclair. Both books have been written by me and will explain in detail the correct way to use your hands for striking and also how to do the named kicks.

Jodan (Upper Body Striking Points)

Tendo *(Crown of the Head)*: This covers the region from the top of the head to the back of the neck. Knife Hand (Shuto), Punch (Tsuki) or Hammer fist (Tetsui) and Elbow Strikes (Empi) are particularly effective in this area.

Tento *(Area between Crown and Forehead)*: Strikes made with hand, elbow and certain foot techniques of potentially lethal effect.

Komekami *(Temple)*: Clearly lethal region particularly susceptible to Tsuki, Tetsui, Shuto or One Knuckle Fist. (Ippon Ken).

Mimi *(Ears)*: Total disorientation and burst ear drums are achieved by attacking both ears with cupped hands. Ears are also susceptible to numerous strikes.

Miken*(Bridge of the Nose)*: Can be classed as potentially lethal by striking the nose with Empi, Shuto,Teisho or Tsuki and various Kicking techniques (Geri waza)

Seidon *(Area Above and Below the Eyes)*: Vulnerable to attack from most Hand Techniques (Te-Waza).

Gansei *(Eyeballs)*: This is one area I leave alone!

Jinchu *(Region Below the Nose)*:Most Te-Waza but specifically Fore knuckle fist (HIRAKEN)
.

Gekon *(Below Lower Lip)*: Again most Te-Waza, but the small hand techniques i.e. Ippon Ken, work the best.

Mikazuki *(Jaw)*: This is one area that you can wallop with most hand and foot techniques with good results.

Dokko *(Behind the Ears)*: Mastoid Process: Susceptible to any point strike (i.e. Ippon Ken, Ippon Nukite etc).

Keichu *(Nape of Neck)*: Again, vulnerable to most Te-waza, hand techniques.

Chudan (Middle Body Striking Points)

Shofu *(Side of Neck)*: Potential lethal strikes are Shuto and Ridgehand strike (Haito uchi)

Sonu *(Base of Throat)*: One-finger piercing strike (Ippon nukite), Two-finger piercing strike (Nihon nukite)

Hichu *(Adam's Apple)*: Most Te Waza but Shuto is extremely good.

Danchu *(Sternum)*: Most Te waza, hand techniques and Geri Waza, foot techniques.

Kyototsu *(Base of Sternum)*: Most Te Waza and Geri Waza.

Suigetsu *(Solar-Plexus)*: Most Te Waza and Geri Waza.

Kyoei *(Below the Armpits)*: Spearhand (Nukite)

Ganchu *(Below the Nipples)*: Most Te Waza and Geri Waza.

Denko *(Between 7th and 8th Ribs)*: Backfist strike, (Uraken)

Inazuma *(Side, Above Hips)*: Most Te Waza

Myojo *(Below Navel)*: Front Kicks using the ball of the foot (Naka-ashi) and most hand techniques

Soda *(Between Shoulder Blades)*: Empi, Shuto and Tetsui are all good strike to this area.

Katsusatsu *(Between 5th and 6th Vertebra)*: Backfist strike, (Uraken) and most small hand techniques

Kodenko *(Base of Spine)*: Certain Geri Waza and most Te Waza.

Wanshun *(Tricep)*: Knife Hand (Shuto), Punch (Tsuki) will cut into this muscle.

Hijizume *(Elbow Joint)*: Attacked with Joint locks.

Udekansetsu *(Arm Joint)*: Attacked with Joint locks.

Kote *(Wrist)*: Attacked with Joint locks.

Uchijakuzawa/Miyakudokoro *(Inside Forearm at Pulse)*: Backfist strike (Uraken) is a clasic strike.

Sotojakuzawa *(Wrist Edge Above Pulse)*: Backfist strike

Shuko *(Back of the Hand)*: Most hand techniques. However if the hand was on the floor holding a weapon you could do a stamping kick (Fumikomi).

Gedan *(Lower Body Striking Points)*

Kinteki *(Testicles)*: Cupped hand, ridge hand, hand flick, knee kick and a good old kick using the top of the foot.

Yako *(Inside Upper Thigh)*: Numerous hand techniques and a round house shin kicks are all powerful to this area.

Fukuto *(Outside Lower Thigh)*: Round house Knee or Shin kick and most punches.

Hizakansetsu *(Knee Joint)*: Front angled kick

Kokotsu *(Inside Shin)*: Front angled kick and most powerful punches

Uchikurobushi *(Inside Ankle Joint)*: Hook kicks and the more powerful hand techniques.

Kori *(Instep)*: Back fist (Uraken) and Empi and Stamp kicks.

Kusagakure *(Outside Top Edge of Foot)*: Empi and most punches and Stamp kicks.

Bitei *(Coccyx)*: Knee Kicks and the more powerful foot and hand techniques

Ushiro-Inazuma *(Below Buttocks)*: Most kicks and most powerful hand techniques are good for this area.

Sobi *(Base of Calf)*: Stamping kick (Fumikomi) and hook kick.

ASHINOYUBI (toes) Stamping kick (Fumikomi).

To sum up Atemi, it is complex system that can take many years of study but it also has some real cool "quick fix techniques" that can be learned in a lesson or two. When reading back over the last sentence, I have realised that this is also the summary for Ju-Jutsu!

I want to move on now to the next range of movements that practised on most Ju-Jutsu classes;

Kansetsu-waza (関節技): Joint locks

Kansetsu-waza is a generic name of joint-locks, which includes fingers, thumbs, wrist, arm, shoulder, leg, foot and neck.

WARNING: Care must be taken when you are applying any joint locking technique. On all Ju-Jutsu classes there is a proper way to submit, tap your partner twice with your hand or tap the mat twice. If for any reason you cannot tap up you say the word 'MATE', it means STOP!

Individual joint-locking techniques are broken down into four categories and have the relevant Japanese names:

Tekubi Kansetsu Waza (wrist-lock techniques)
Ude Kansetsu Waza (arm-lock techniques)
Ashi Kansetsu Waza (leg-lock techniques)
Kubi Kansetsu Waza (neck-lock techniques)

These four categories can be broken down further into two groups, according to technique which follows joint-locking.

Kansetsu-waza for Nage-waza (throwing techniques)
Kansetsu-waza for Katame-waza (holding techniques)

What is a Joint lock?

A joint lock is a grappling technique involving the manipulation of an opponent's joints in such a way that the joints reach their maximal degree of motion. These typically involve isolating a particular joint, and leveraging it in an attempt to force the joint to move past its normal range of motion. Joint locks usually involve varying degrees of pain in the joints, and if applied forcefully and/or suddenly, may cause injury, such as muscle, tendon and ligament damage, even dislocation, or bone fractures.

Some joint locks such as an elbow are extremely easy to apply with extremely painful result; this is because the principle used is a lever and fulcrum.

What is a lever and fulcrum?

To under stand this we have to look to elementary physics. I know that you are now thinking of "flipping a few pages" as the thought in your head must be "Doesn't this Ju-Jutsu get complicated" But please be patient, once you understand this simple process, you will be able to apply locks on people who are a lot bigger and stronger than your are with little strength and extremely painful results. So let's plod on; there are three types of levers: 1st Class, 2nd Class, and 3rd Class. The relative position of the load, fulcrum and force determine the class of lever. What I am about to describe in martial arts is a 1st class lever. This is a very common lever that is utilised in many Ju-Jutsu joint locking techniques.

In martial arts terms the lever is the limb you intend to apply the lock on. In this case we are looking at an elbow lock so you would take a hold of the arm just above the wrist joint. What you need now is a fulcrum; this will be your other arm. Place this arm just above the just above the elbow joint of the arm you are holding. Now you have pivot point to make the lever work. Keep the "fulcrum arm still" and with the hand that is on the wrist apply a little pressure so the elbow joint becomes locked. You will hardy need any strength as the lock comes on very easily. Apply more pressure and you could easily snap an elbow joint!

I know this is a little complicated so in illustration 3, a. I have applied a class 1 lever "elbow lock" on one of my student's right arms so you can see exactly what I mean. The red arrows indicate the lever, fulcrum and pressure being applied. In this illustration, I have hooked my left arm under the attacker's right arm and am using my left bicep as the fulcrum. The pressure to apply the elbow lock is been done with my right hand pushing down at the attackers right wrist.

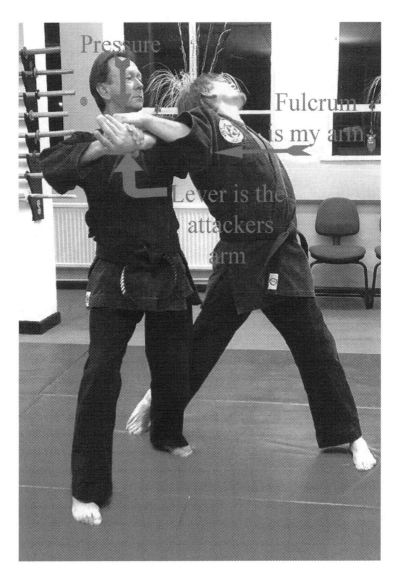

Illustration 3, a.

Fulcrums can be applied with different parts of the body. In illustration 4, a, I am still using the attacker's right arm as the lever, but this time I am using my upper thigh as the fulcrum. The right hand on the wrist is pushing down and is applying the pressure. To make the lever more stable, I have taken a hold of the attacker's lapel, this stretches his right arm out more so the lock is then easier to apply.

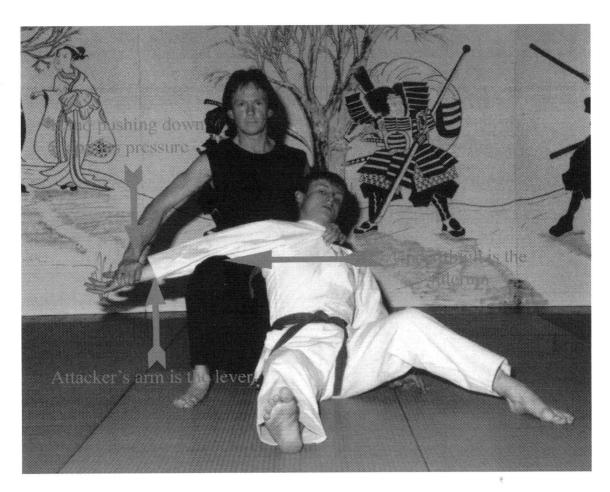

Illustration 4, a.

Ok, you may have noticed that this is an "old picture" of me. Well the reason I wanted to put this in is to show you that hair fashions change. We all get older. And over the years that I have been practising martial arts, the arts have gone go through different trends, kick boxing, tai bo and so on. But a lock is a lock no matter how old it is and the principles of applying a lock will never change.

One thing that must be noted is that Ju-Jutsu is very resourceful when it comes to elbow locks and indeed any other lock. In illustration 6, a, (another old photo) I have applied an elbow lock to the attacker's right arm using the back of my left calf muscle as the fulcrum. The attacker's right arm is the lever and to compound the pain that he is getting. Using my right hand I have applied a wrist lock to the attacker's right wrist joint.

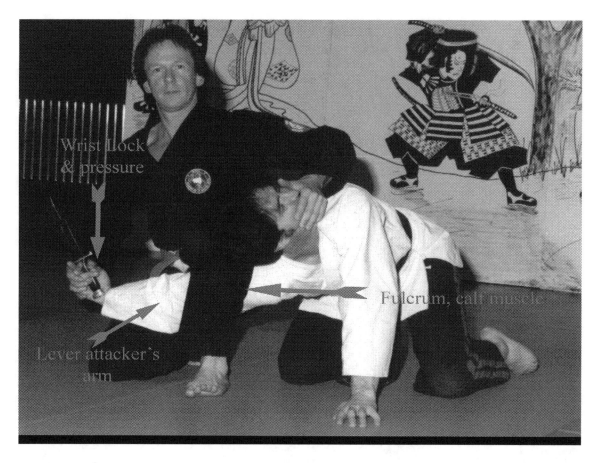

Labels on image: "Wrist lock & pressure", "Lever attacker's arm", "Fulcrum, calf muscle"

Illustration 6, a.

As you can see from illustration 6, a, I have placed my left hand across the attackers Jaw and mouth, the hand on the jaw helps stretch out the attackers upper body and the hand across his mouth stops him screaming in pain!!!!

Now I have a little test for you. Let's see if you have grasped the basics of a 1st class lever. Look at illustration 7, a, and see if you can determine the following;

What part of the attacker's body is the lever? What part of the body is being used as a fulcrum? What is being used to exert the pressure? And finally I have included in illustration 7, a, a small diagram in the bottom right hand corner of a fulcrum, lever, force and load. The question is, what would represent the "load" in illustration 7, a?

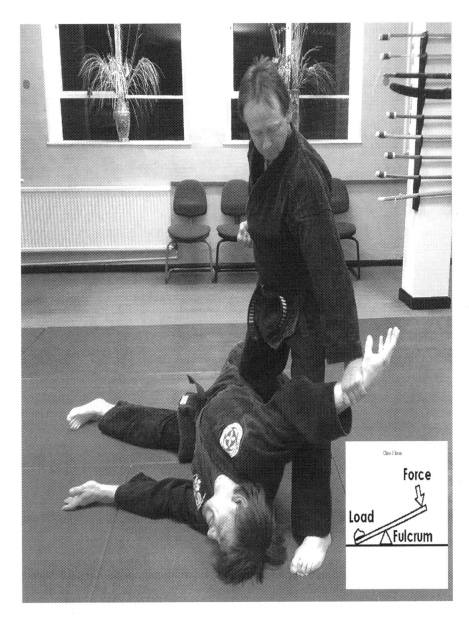

Illustration 7, a.

Technically speaking, Ude Kansetsu Waza (arm-lock techniques) could also be called Hiji Kansetsu Waza (elbow-lock techniques) As in most cases it is the elbow that is being locked.

How many Kansetsu Waza (Joint locking techniques) are there in Ju-Jutsu?

I will answer this question with another question, how many stars are there in the known universe? That will give you some idea of how many locking techniques and locking variations there are in Ju-Jutsu. Every joint in your body can be manipulated into locking techniques and this can be done while you are standing, sitting, against a wall, belly down on the floor, on your side or flat on your back.

Not only can you apply a locking techniques to one joint, you can also apply locks to two or more joints. In illustration 7, a, (Another old, old photo) I have my opponent on the floor, face down and am applying a "double wrist and double shoulder lock".

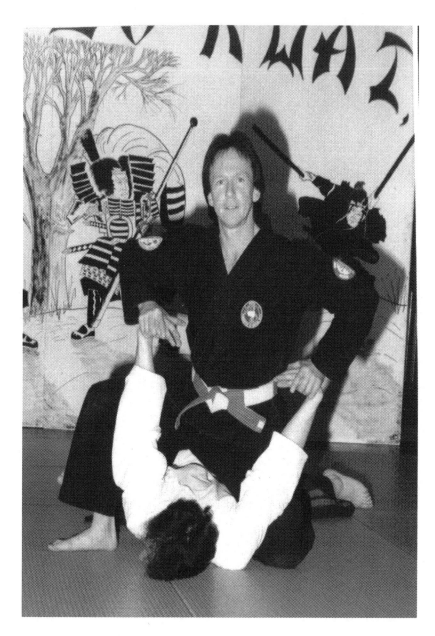

Illustration 7, a.

I want to conclude this brief explanation of Kansetsu Waza (joint locking techniques) by showing you one more "Old" illustration. In illustration 8, a, I have my opponent on his side and I am applying an elbow lock to his right elbow (using a 1st class lever) and a wrist lock to his left wrist. This would be classed as a "combination joint locking technique" as I am applying two completely different joint locking techniques.

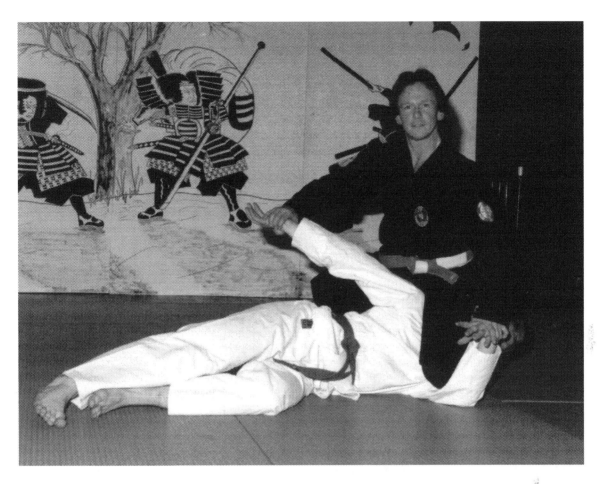

Illustration 8, a.

Nage-waza, 投げ技, throwing techniques.

The next thing you can expect to learn on a Ju-Jutsu class is, Nage-waza, (投げ技), throwing techniques.

So what is a throw?

A throw is where you unbalance your adversary by one of several Ju-Jutsu unbalancing methods and then proceed to throw or forcibly project them to the floor or into or onto objects that may be in the immediate vicinity.

When you first start on a Ju-Jutsu class, the throws you can expect to do are very basic. This is due to the fact that safety comes first, you have to learn how to breakfall safely and also know how to control your training partner whilst throwing them. Once those factors are out of the way, Ju-Jutsu has hundreds of throwing techniques, some are Judo based throws, others will be Aiki based throws and then you have the "Ju-Jutsu exclusive" throws.

Nage Waza (throwing techniques) are broken down in to the following categories; Hand techniques, Shoulder techniques, Hip techniques, Neck techniques, Leg techniques, Front throws (throwing the person face down), Back throws (throwing the person onto there back) Side throws (throwing the person onto there side, Rear sacrifice throws (this is where the thrower drops to the floor onto his or her back and throws his opponent) Side sacrifice throws (this is where the thrower drops to the floor on his or her side and throws his opponent. And (advanced students only) reverse throws, (this is where you throw someone from front to back or vice versa).

From a Ju-Jutsu prospective the scope of throwing techniques is vast. In addition to the above, you can do aikido related throws, floor throws (that is where you are actually lying on the floor) and throws off various kicks, the list is almost infinite.

The key to any throw is getting your opponent off balance. The methodology used in Ju-Jutsu varies according to the type of attack and can often be a simple atemi (strike), a pull, push or an intricate lock that leads into a throw.

In Japanese terms unbalancing is called Kuzushi (崩し：くずし) however there are two other components that make for a successful throw, Tsukuri (meaning entering) and Kake (meaning the final execution of the throw).

These three words, Kuzushi, Tsukuri and Kake have been debated by Scholars and experts from many throwing arts and have all come up with various theories on the exact meaning of each word. I have my own explanation which I feel sums up each word simply; Kuzushi is the most important factor as this is the start of the throw as this is how you draw the attacker off balance, so I simply call this the "Start". Once you have the "start" correct, you can now move to the next phase, Tsukuri is how you enter and align yourself in readiness for the throw, this is the what I call the "Middle" of the throw. Kake is the execution and end of the throw. So I call this the "End". To sum up, if you get the "start", "middle" and "end" right you have just pulled off the perfect throw.

I know that I have over simplified the whole theory behind getting an opponent off balance, but in my 'books'……… why make a mountain out of a mole hill?

To help you visualize unbalancing principles, I have chosen the next three illustrations that will show you the basic principles of getting someone off balance using a typical Judo grip and then throwing them using a throw is known as a major hip throw (O Goshi).

In illustration 9 a, I have taken a hold of my practice partners jacket. My right hand has taken a grip of the outside of his left lapel and my left hand has taken a grip of his right jacket sleeve.

With a good firm grip, I draw my partner off balance by pulling upward in a small arc. This results in my partner being lifted up so that his body weight goes into his toes and his heels are lifted of the floor or mats.

The idea behind this is to raise my partner's centre of balance; an easy indicator is look at your partner's belt, it should be a few inches above your own. This now make him top heavy, this can be seen in illustration 9 a. The result of unbalancing him using this method is it makes my entry into the throw easy. This is called Kuzushi (the start).

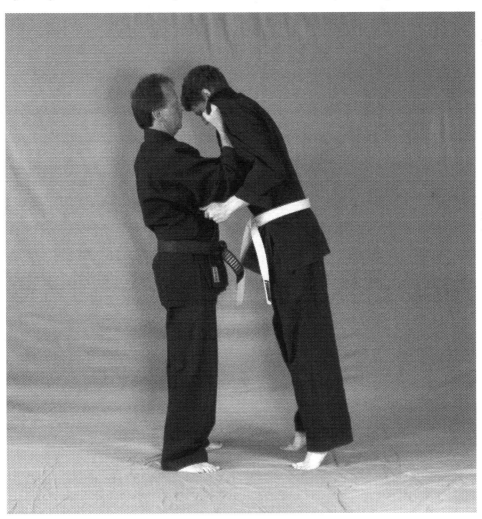

Illustration 9 a, (Kuzushi) the start.

With my partner off balance, I have swiftly moved in and lifted him up using the major hip throw lifting method. He is now balanced precisely on my right hip in a sea saw position. It is surprising how easy this is once you have the lifting and balance method correct.

If you wish to practice this, I would recommend that you only do this in a safe environment for example at a DOJO where someone with the expertise is able to advise you on the correct procedure for the lift onto the hip.

Illustration 9 b, shows my partner being lifted onto my right hip in preparation to being thrown. As this is the middle of the technique it is classed as Tsukuri (the middle).

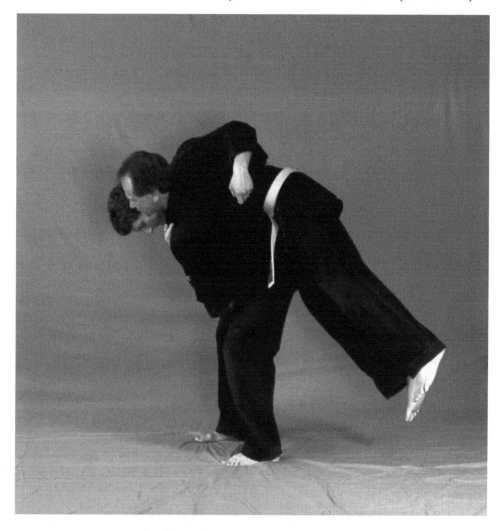

Illustration 9 b, (Tsukuri) the middle.

From illustration 9 b, I turn my head from right to left and at the same time I draw my partner across my body by pulling from right to left. This results in my partner been thrown to the floor/mats. This is the final execution of the throw and is called Kake (the end).

Illustration 9,c shows the completion of the major hip throw O Goshi.

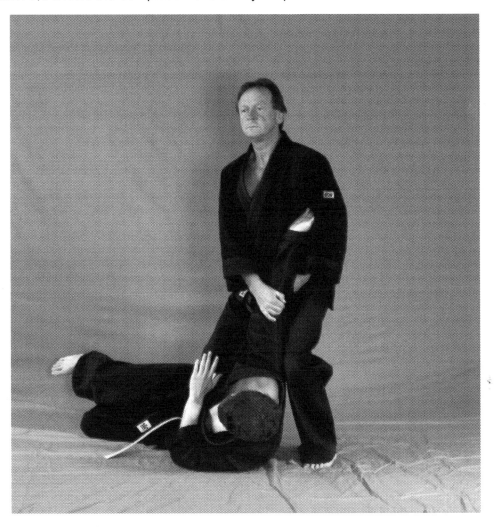

Illustration 9, c, Kake, the end.

The next section will be dedicated to showing various Ju-Jutsu throws from various attacks. This is where Ju-Jutsu excels as a self defence art; numerous skills will now be employed in order to successfully execute the throwing technique. Just remember that in all throws, you have to get the attacker off balance.

I will explain each throw with enough detail so that you the reader can then practice these techniques. Before you consider doing this, you must think of your own personal safety. Only practice in a proper Dojo that has a Tatami (mat area). If you are inexperienced, seek the assistance from a Sensei (teacher) or other high graded martial artist.

For those who have more Ju-Jutsu knowledge, you can always enhance the following throws with some spectacular locks, strangulation and immobilisation techniques.

YOUR HOME, GARDEN and BACK YARD ARE NOT A SAFE PLACE TO PRACTICE JU-JUTSU OR ANY OTHER MARTIAL ART.

In all of the techniques I demonstrate in this book, I will only show them on side. Remember when you practice them get familiar with one side and then have a go on the opposite side.

Front strangulation into a major hip throw.

O Goshi (大腰) English aliases: Major Hip (Roll) Throw, Large Hip Throw

In illustration 10 a, the attacker has lunged forward and is strangling me with both hands around my neck. Before I can attempt to do any defensive techniques, I need to gain and maintain my own balance. Part of learning how to defend oneself is understanding the mechanics of the attack. In this instance the attacker has lunged at me with both hands directed towards my neck. Consequently this has thrown me off balance and in order to regain my balance I have had to adjust my body posture. For this, I have brought my left leg forward and now have a left posture. The white arrow in illustration 10 a, indicates that I have stepped forward with my left leg to maintain my balance and posture.

For those who are new to martial arts, you must try not to panic or struggle in any attack situation, sadly, panic only makes the attack worse for you and easier for the attacker. You may now be thinking "how the hell do I not panic when someone is trying to kill me by strangling me?" Well the answer is; you must get used of being attacked. Every newcomer starts Ju-Jutsu with gentle practice, but then the intensity of the practice and attacks should increase as you become more proficient with your techniques.

The idea behind this is you are so familiar with being attacked that you automatically respond with the appropriate defence and do not go into shock. Shock is an attacker's best friend. The attacker instinctively knows that shock will set in immediately from the onset of an attack and is relying on its effects so that you will be unable to defend yourself.

When I teach my students defences from this kind of attack, I often introduce a little reverse psychology. In this particular attack where the attacker has both hands around the neck, I teach that the attacker has tied up two of his major weapons and therefore the attack is not as bad as it first seems. If we changed this attack scenario and the attacker was grasping my neck with one hand and firing punches into my face with the other free hand, then the attack/defence would be more challenging. So now the two handed strangulation isn't that bad.

I also teach PMA, this stands for **positive mental attitude** and that's what you must always have. Thinking positively will make you a winner not just in an attack situation but also in life. Thinking negatively about anything will always produce negative results; with my reverse psychology and PMA, we can always turn a negative into a positive.

Illustration 10 a, shows the attackers attempting to strangle me, I my first line of defence is gaining my balance.

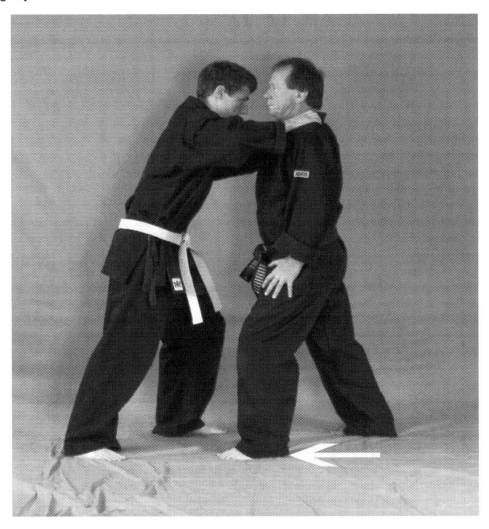

Illustration 10, a.

Now that I stabilized my posture, I can start with my opening movements and they come in a neat package of three simultaneous movements. This may be a little complicated to start, but it gets easier with practice............OK......... lots of practice, but that what martial arts is all about.

I step with the right leg so that it is aligned with the centre of the attacker's body. At the same time my left hands rises up and grasps the attacker's inside right arm, just above the wrist and I simultaneously fire a jab out with my right fist striking the attacker in his stomach. The jab, Atemi momentarily stuns the attacker and that allows me to pull his right hand away from my throat.

Illustration 10 b shows all three simultaneous movements with two added guide arrows. The arrow on the floor shows the direction I step with my right foot and the other arrow shows the right fist jabbing, using an Atemi into the attacker's stomach.

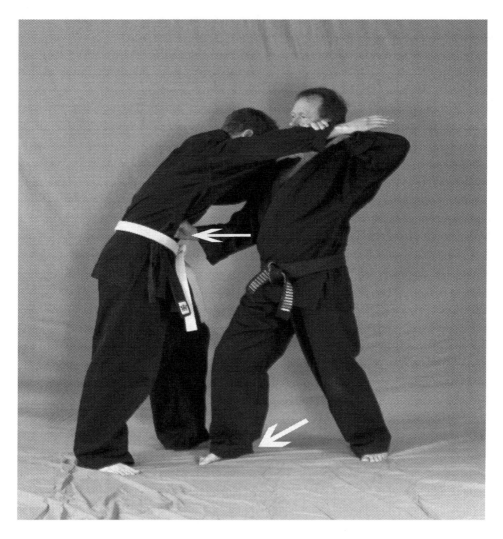

Illustration 10 b.

Whilst the attacker is momentarily stunned from the jab Atemi to the stomach, I need to do a few more simultaneous movements to get myself into a throwing position.

I have pivoted on the right foot so that I am almost facing the same direction as the attacker. At the same time I reverse my left leg back, this aligns my body so now my hips are tucked just below the attacker's waist line, my partner now becomes top heavy and that is the advantage I need to be able to be able to throw him.

I am quite fortunate in this routine as my attacker is taller than I am. This means I have not had to bend my knees to much in order to lower my posture to get myself below his centre of balance. It will be completely different for you........... **Attacker's come in all shapes and sizes.** If you are practising this movement, it will be necessary to bend your knees in order to compensate for the attacker's or practice partner's size. A simple gauge is to make sure your belt line is below that of your partners or attackers belt line. Tall people always have to work harder at throwing a smaller person as they have to bend there knees more to get below the centre of gravity when entering a throwing technique. When the role is reversed, the shorter person throwing a taller person has a distinct advantage.

As I reverse my left foot back, I simultaneously reach around the attacker's waist with my right arm and pull the attacker tight into my body. The curved arrow in illustration 10 c shows where my right arm has travelled from and where my right hand is gripping just above the attacker's waist line.

My left hand still maintains the grip on the attack's right wrist keeping the attacker's arm in an elevated position. I have used a white arrow pointing upwards to show this in illustration 10 c. This arm position is crucial to that unbalancing and intimately the throwing of the attacker as it acts as a counter lever.

Illustration 10 c, shows all of the above, study this illustration and then try to replicate the movements.

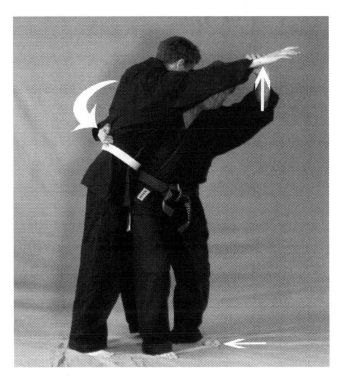

Illustration 10 c.

Next, I pull down sharply with my left hand and simultaneously bend my knees and tilt my body forward, this draws the attacker off balance to the point where I can easily lift him. The attacker is now balanced on my hips with his feet off the floor or mats.

This is shown in illustration 10.d. The white arrow in this illustration indicates the direction I have used to pull downward with my left hand.

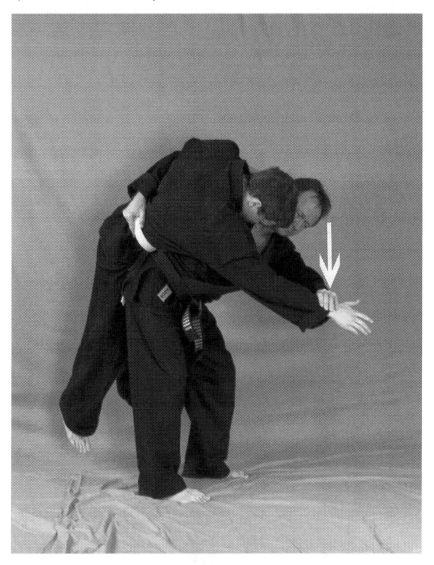

Illustration 10.d.

I now continue with the throwing action by pulling my left arm to my left side and also rotating my body in the same direction.

It is important to keep both feet flat on the floor when throwing somebody as it helps maintain your own balance and the decisive control of the attacker. At this stage, I have had to make a small stepping adjustment with my right foot to compensate for my balance and control of the attacker's body while he is in flight. I am now in the ideal throwing position with both my feet level and placed just underneath my hips.

The curved white arrow in illustration 10 e shows the direction that I use in order to continue throwing the attacker.

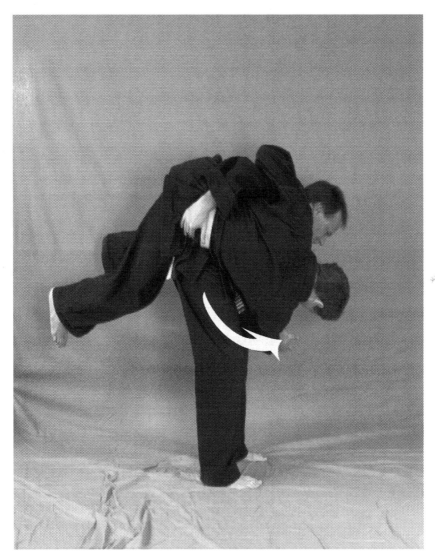

Illustration 10 e.

I have now passed the point of no return and the attacker is thrown to the floor......or in my case the mats.

Even after you throw someone hard to the floor they may still be able to fight back due to the effects following; drugs, alcohol and a natural substance, adrenalin. I have automatically anticipated this and have kept control of the attacker's right arm by maintaining my grip with my left hand; this has left the attacker's right side open.

Illustration 10, f shows the attacker on the floor and my right fist ready to strike the attacker.

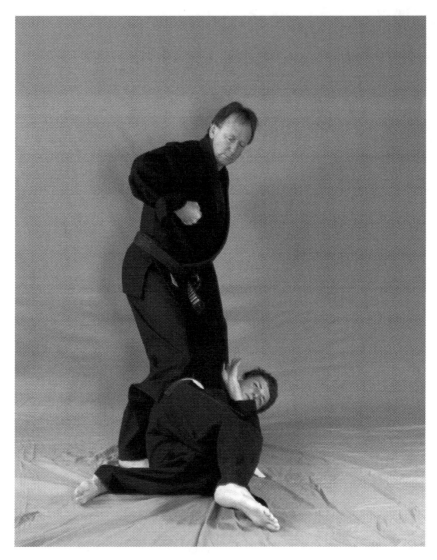

To finalise this throwing routine, I have dropped into a lower forward stance and delivered a powerful punch to the attacker's right rib area using my right fist. This is shown in illustration 10, g. To enhance the power of the final punch or indeed any punch or strike, you can add a Kiai (martial battle cry).

If I were doing this or any other defensive technique from a real attack in the street, I would take a fighting stance immediately after the final blow in readiness for any other potential attacker's. It is always better to be safe than sorry.

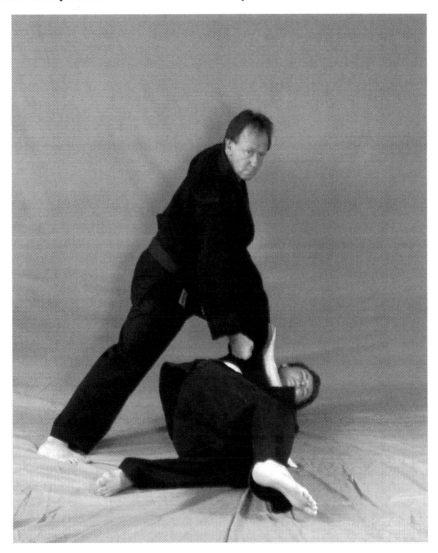

Illustration 10 ,g.

This concludes the front strangulation into a major hip throw routine, I know you will be keen to try out this throwing routine, just remember to practice right and left.

Downward blow to the head and one arm shoulder throw

(Ippon Seoinage). (一本 背負投) English Aliases: One arm shoulder throw ,diagonal throw

As this is an extremely serious attack from a street point of view, you have a number of options:

Run away, this on face value might sound strange, but it is a serious option that could ultimately save your life. No one is a coward for recognising a bad situation and living through it. Martial arts are all about survival. In the Dojo there are no rules that state that once you learn a few techniques, you have to stand and fight. On the contrary, you will find that the more you learn about Ju-Jutsu the less you will want to fight. Why? Because the technique are extremely effective..................This is not an ambiguous statement, it is a fact of life................... or indeed .... Death, especially if you are the attacker!

Comply; the attacker could be a mugger who is demanding cash or other items. You and you alone have to make a conscious decision as to stand and fight or hand over the cash. Before you snap at me saying "they can have my cash......Ha.... over my dead body" Life has a way of complicating things. What would you do if you were with your family, put them in unnecessary danger? What if the attacker has some armed companions? These complications are not a fantasy; they are what could happen in the real world, as a martial artist you have to be able to adjust to each situation. Complying sometimes is the only option.

Utilise items that are available to assist in your defence. For example, if the attack were in your home, a small chair could be used to throw at the attacker; an arm chair could be used as an obstacle to block the attacker's path. It is said that an "English mans home is his castle" It can also be said "every home is an armoury" if you just open your eyes. This is true of every where you go; natural weapons are always at hand, just start looking.

Carry a weapon? This is not an option, just a simple warning. **If you carry a weapon, you will use it.** Regrettably many of us feel that society has let us down and the streets are lawless. Knife and gun crime are not just a daily occurrence, these crimes happen every few seconds! The temptation for individuals to arm themselves for self defence purposes is indeed understandable, but it is not the answer. Laws need to be tightened; prison sentencing needs to be stiffer and certain people's attitude towards a communal society as a whole needs to be seriously addressed. All of this will not happen over night. I personally fear things will only get worse! The problem is that if you carry a weapon, you have already shown a degree of intention and that weighs heavy in the eyes of the law. Add to this the usage of the said weapon and you are now in serious trouble. You could end up killing someone and spending many precious years of your life behind bars when all you had to do was run away or comply. Ok, I think it is time for some PMA (positive mental attitude). Martial arts equips you with all the weapons you need, in each hand you have a minimum thirty two weapons, that sixty four using both hands. Add all the kicks, throws, locks, strangulation techniques and immobilisation techniques and you are now a walking munitions store. So do you really need to carry a weapon?

Defend oneself; I strongly recommend that this option is one that must be taken deadly serious! Be prepared to explore every possible attack scenario and work on the defence of that attack until you become highly competent and then move on to the next one. As there are hundreds of thousands of different ways of being attacked this should take you a life time.

The attacker for this routine is armed with a cosh in his right hand; he has already raised it up showing that his intention is to attack my head area. In readiness for the attack, I have come into a left fighting stance. This is shown in illustration 11,a.

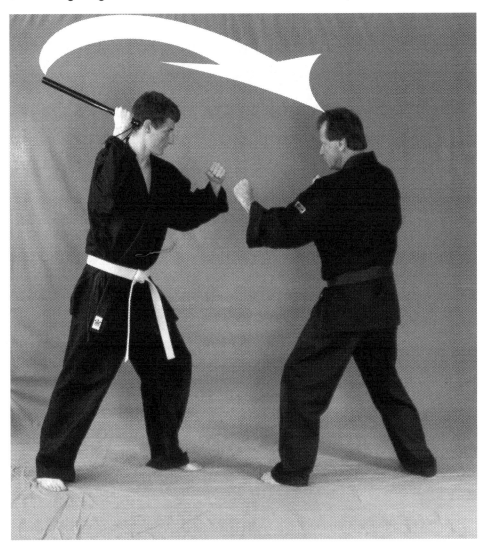

Illustration 11, a.

Trying to cave my skull in with the cosh, the attacker swings a powerful blow to my head. From my left fighting stance, I extend my left leg forward into a left forward stance. At the same time I use my left arm to block strike the attacker's right arm, just above his wrist joint. Block striking is a technique I favour; it allows me to power through an attacker's arm, causing him immense pain through the striking impact.

Illustration 11, b shows the attacker's cosh arm being driven back with my powerful block strike, the white curved arrow shows the direction that my left arm has travelled in. The white arrow on the floor shows how I have stepped in order to take a powerful left forward stance.

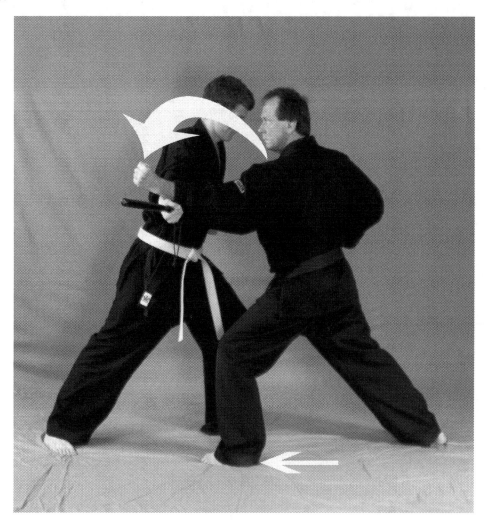

Illustration 11, b.

As the block strike reaches its completion, I use my left hand and grasp hold of the attacker's right wrist. In a simultaneous movement, my right fist strikes, Atemi the attacker's sternum or breast bone, this makes him jerk back from his upper torso. This is an important strike, Atemi as it sets the attacker up for the one arm shoulder throw. How so? Well, it keeps the attacker's posture upright and that helps my entry into this particular throw. If I had struck the attacker in the groin he would now be bending forward and with that body posture, it would make the one arm shoulder throw almost impossible! The moral of this is you must match your strikes, Atemi with the throws you are doing.

Illustration 11, c has two arrows on it; one shows my left hand grasping the attacker's right wrist. The other shows my right hand striking, Atemi the attacker's sternum or breast bone.

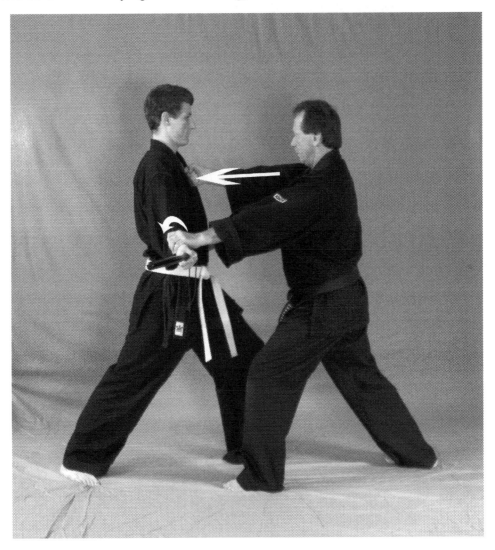

Illustration 11, c.

As soon as the strike, Atemi has landed, I step across with my right foot so that it is pointing towards the attacker's right foot. This is shown in illustration, d. The white arrow on the floor in the same illustration shows the direction that I have stepped in.

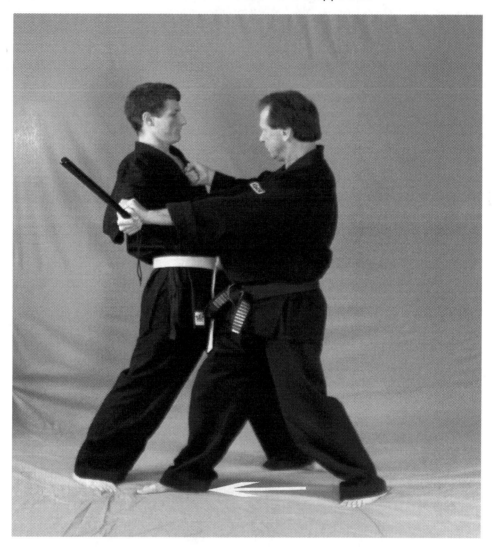

Illustration 11, d.

I maintain my grip with my left hand and quickly pass my right arm under the attacker's right arm. As I do this, I grab the cloth of his jacket with my right hand. If you were doing this out in the street and the attacker is not wearing a jacket...........No problem, just grab a hold of his or her arm.

At the same time, I have reversed my left leg backward, tucked my hips in, just a tad deeper than in the major hip throw and then pulled sharply forward with my right and left hand. The result is, I now have the attacker off balance and have been able to have lift the attacker up in readiness for the throw. He is now balancing on my right hip and is aligned to be thrown over my right shoulder. Note; my feet are pointing in the same direction and directly under my hips for balance and control.

Illustration 11, e shows the attacker half way through the one arm shoulder throw. The white arrow on the floor shows that my left leg has reversed, aligning me correctly for the throw.

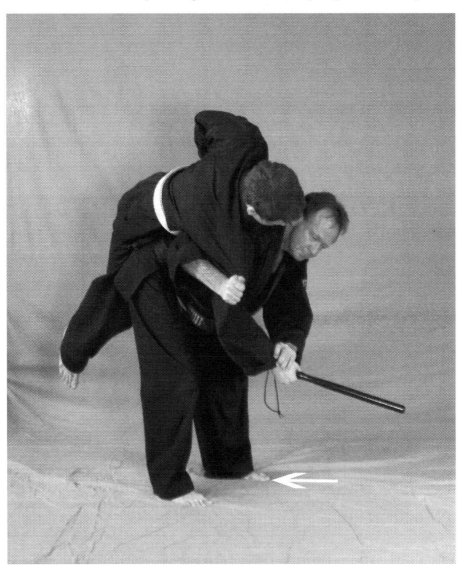

Illustration 11 e.

The throw is achieved about a millisecond later by drawing the attacker's body from my right to my left.

It is important to maintain control of the attacker's right arm. I do this by keeping a hold of it with my left hand. As soon as he hit the mats, floor. I use my left hand to pull his right arm upward sharply to my left side. This helps throw the attacker on his side, the result of this is: It minimises fight back with the attacker's left hand and also exposes his right rib area.

Illustration 11, f shows the attacker thrown to the mats, floor. With me hovering, ready to deliver a strike to his right rib area with my right fist.

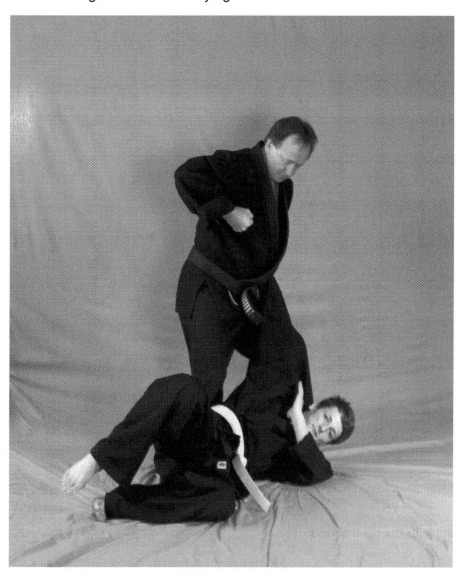

Illustration 11, f.

I finalize this throwing routine by dropping into a forward stance and striking the attacker in the ribs with my right fist. Just for extra control, I have placed the attacker's right elbow joint onto my inner thigh and by pushing downward with my right hand. I have an elbow lock on the attacker. This is shown in Illustration 11, g.

At this stage, if the attacker is still holding the weapon, I would in a strong voice tell him **"let the weapon go"** If he was stupid enough to try to hold onto the weapon, I would apply more pressure on the elbow lock and then repeat my verbal command. If this were a real attack, I would be prepared to break the attacker's elbow if he didn't comply with my verbal commands. This is where you have to realise Ju-Jutsu is not a game, it is an effective method of self defence and self preservation.

Once I complete a defence where a weapon is involved, I always retrieve the weapon so that it cannot be used again.

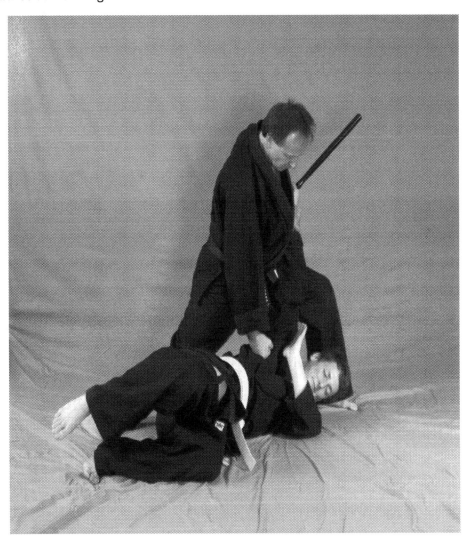

Illustration 11, g.

This concludes the attack from a downward blow into a one arm should throw. Don't forget to practice this routine right and left and add a kiai for more power when you punch.

Low side blow into neck throw....Body drop style.
Kubi Nage, also known as Koshi Guruma, (腰車)

Ju-Jutsu throwing techniques are not identical to those found in Judo (sports style) or pure Aiki-do. They are rough diamonds ready to be cut and shaped as the need arises. The next throw is typical of this, its a bit of a mongrel; it starts out as a neck throw, (Kubi Nage, also known as Koshi Guruma) (腰車), and ends up as neck throw using the body drop principle.

In illustration 12 a, the attacker has squared up to me and we are both in a fighting stance, left legs forward.

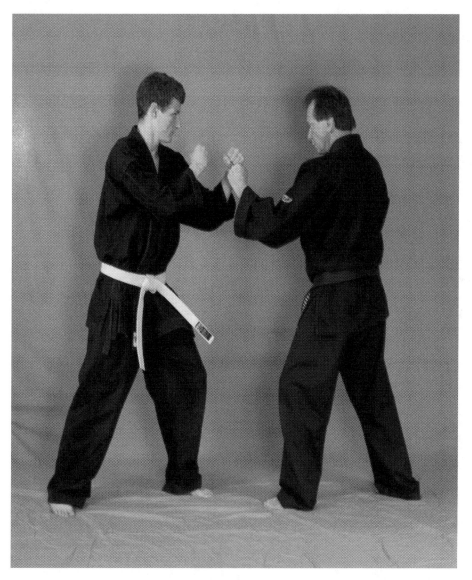

The attacker steps forward with his left leg and fires a low blow out with his right fist. His intention is; get to get below my guard position and roundhouse punch me in the ribs.

To counter this attack, I step away from him with my right foot into an offset forward stance; this takes my body offline from the low roundhouse blow. In the same motion as the step, I use my left outside forearm and downward block strike the attackers left inside forearm. The principle of this block is to stop the attacker's left hand before it passes his own left shoulder. It's amazing how weak the blow is at this point. The timing of the block is critical. If you are practicing this block, do not let the attacker's hand travel any further than I have described as you will have difficulty stopping the attack.

Illustration 12, b shows the attacker arm being blocked by my downward outside forearm block strike. The curved white arrow shows the direction the attacker throws his low roundhouse punch, while the white arrow on the floor shows the direction I have stepped with my right foot to achieve my offset forward stance.

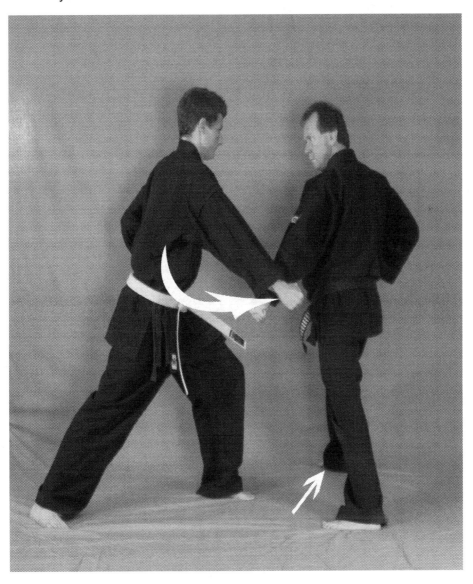

Illustration 12, b.

In one smooth powerful action, by pivoting on the ball of my feet. I switch my body weight from my right forward stance to a left forward stance.

At the same time, I swing my right arm in an arc, striking the attacker on the side of the neck with my right inside forearm, this is an Atemi. The result of this strike is; it throws the attacker off balance…... (Scrambles his brain) and lowers his head. This is exactly what I wanted to achieve, as I intend to place my right arm around the back of his neck.

Illustration 12, c shows the attacker been struck with my right inside forearm strike, the white curved arrow shows the direction my right arm has travelled in. The lower white arrow shows the change in direction of my stance.

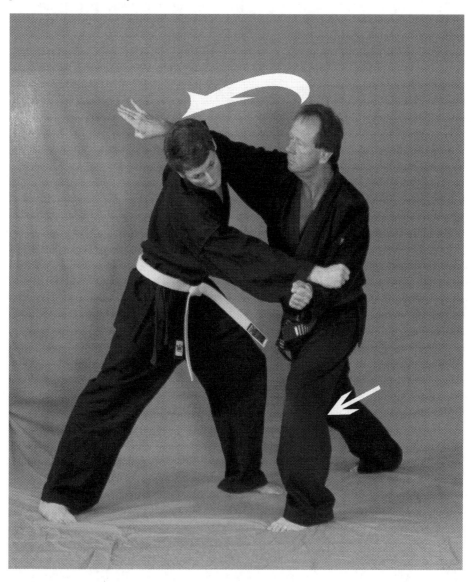

Illustration 12, c.

Now that I have stunned the attacker, I instantly wrap my right arm around the attacker's neck and grab a hold of the attacker's right shoulder with my right hand. At the same time, I have grabbed a hold of the attacker's right sleeve with my left hand and pull this in tightly to my body. I have additionally reversed my feet and tucked my hips in deeply so that both my feet are under my hips.

The attacker's centre of balance is very low due to the neck strike knocking him forward; this makes me have to squat very low as I enter into the throwing position.

Illustration 12, d shows my right arm around the attacker's neck, my left hand pulling the attack's right arm tight into my body and my hips tucked in to the attacker's body. The white arrows should help guide you through the above movements.

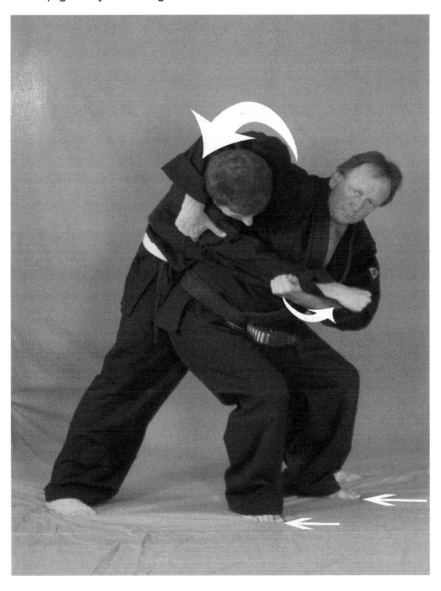

Illustration 12, d.

To achieve a lift to throw in my current position would be extremely difficult; this is due to the attacker's body weight pushing down onto my hips. To compensate for this, I shoot my right leg out to my right side, placing my right foot outside of the attacker's right foot. This movement has now lowered my body satisfactorily and I am now well below the attacker's centre of balance.

Illustration 12, e shows a white arrow pointing in the direction I have moved my right leg. Note; I have a small bend in my right knee and that I am balancing on the ball of my right foot; this will help give me upward spring, when I am throwing the attacker.

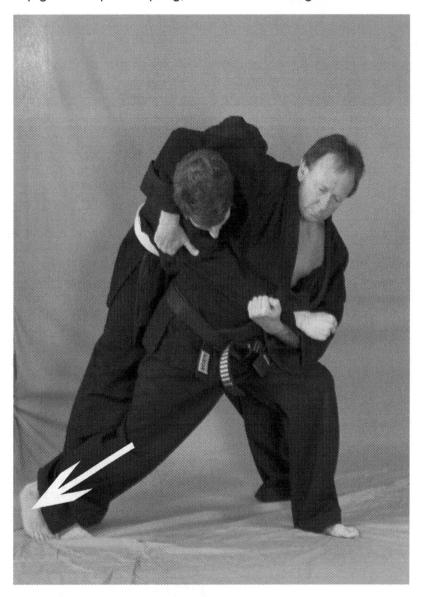

Illustration 12, e.

I now push upwards with my hips; at the same time, I straighten my right leg and flatten my right foot to the floor. These actions literally spring the attacker's body up and off balance. As I feel the attacker's feet leave the floor or mats, I pull sharply from right to left with both arms and at the same time I turn my body in the same direction. This now has the attacker in flight and being thrown towards the floor or mats.

Illustration 12, f shows the attacker half way through the throw, the white curved arrow shows the direction I am pulling him in so that I can complete the throw.

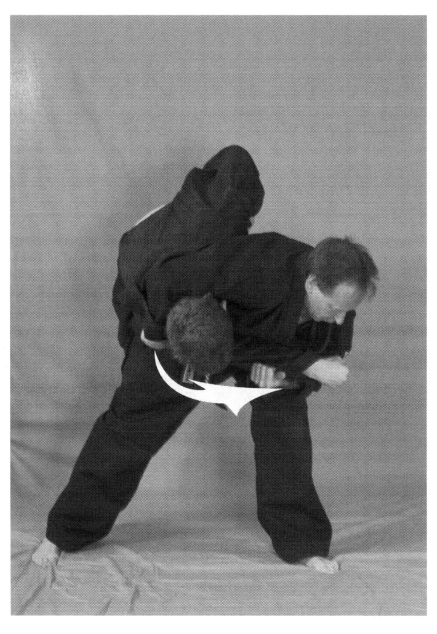

Illustration 12, f.

As the attacker's body drops to the floor, I instantly drop down on my right knee; this adds more impact to the throw. To maintain my balance, I have kept my right knee up in a kneeling stance.

To finalize this throwing routine, I have kept control of the attacker's right arm with my left hand and in simultaneous movements: I apply and elbow lock to the attack's right elbow by placing the elbow joint on my inner thigh and then pushing down with my left hand. This stretches out the attacker's upper torso, making the ribs extremely vulnerable. I take full advantage of this, by striking the attacker's ribs with my left fist, this is an Atemi. A kiai at this stage would add lots more power.

Illustration 12, g shows the finish to the low side blow into neck throw....Body drop style.

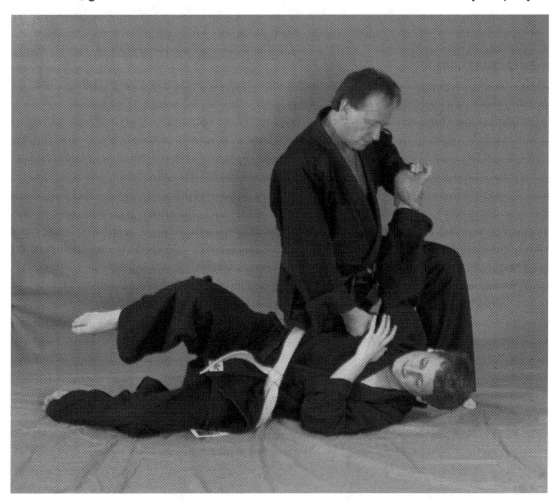

Illustration 12, g.

Before you practice this routine, **warn your partner,** that the breakfall from this throw is, **extremely heavy,** due to the fact that you drop to one knee as your partner falls towards the mats.

Don't forget to practice this routine on the other side.

Two fast round house punches into a Lifting Pulling Ankle Block, Ju-Jutsu style.

For the next throwing routine, I want to demonstrate a Lifting Pulling Ankle Block, (Sasae Tsurikomi Ashi) (支釣込足) English Aliases: Propping & Drawing Ankle Throw, Stopping Foot Throw or Stopping Leg Throw.

The attacker has come into a fighting stance, left leg forward, with his guard up. In anticipation of any potential attack, I have also come into a fighting stance, left leg forward, with my guard up. This is shown in illustration 13, a.

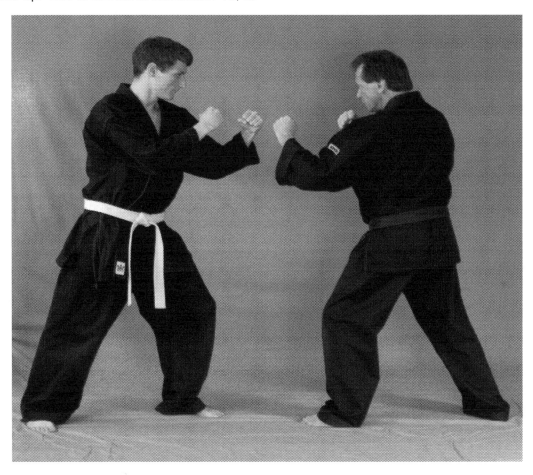

Illustration 13, a.

The attacker decides to go for it; he lunges at me with a left round house punch to my head. To make up the distance between us, he has also had to step forward with his left leg.

To counter this attack, I keep my left leg forward, drop quickly into a forward stance and use a reverse outside forearm block strike. This stops the attackers arm well before he has a chance to strike me. The attacker also feels as if he has just thrown his arm, full force at a solid tree trunk! Now that's a bonus for me........and you, if you utilize the same blocking methods.

Illustration 13, b shows the attacker's arm being blocked by my reverse outside forearm block. The white curved arrow shows the direction the attacker has swung his blow at me.

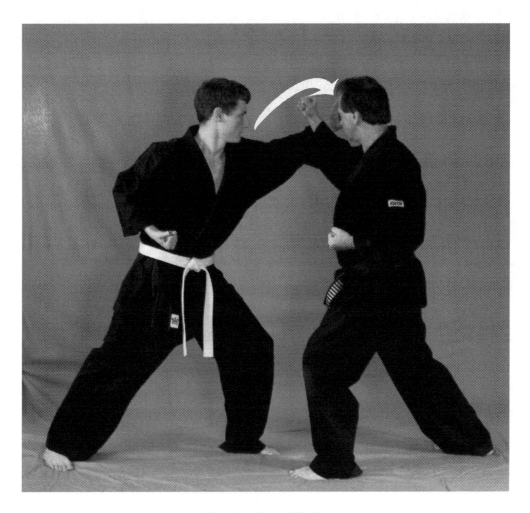

Illustration 13, b.

In less than a blink of an eye, the attacker fires another roundhouse punch to my head! This time he uses his right fist.

My counter has to be fast! I switch my stance immediately by stepping away from the attacker with my right foot. This take my head offline from the roundhouse punch, it also gets my into a strong forward stance with my right foot forward. In a simultaneous movement, I reverse block strike the attacker's right arm with my left outside forearm.

By now, the attacker's left and right inside forearms should be deadened from the severe impacts from my block strikes!

Illustration 13, c shows me countering the attacker roundhouse punch with a reverse outside forearm block. The curved white arrow shows the direction of the attacker's roundhouse punch.

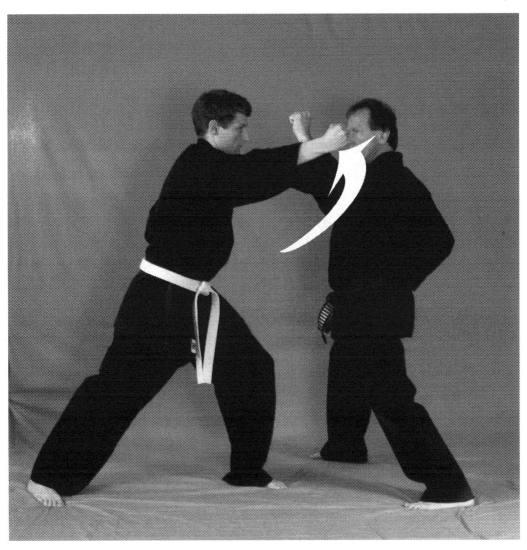

Illustration 13, c.

In preparing to throw an attacker, you have to identify the exact position at which he or she is off balance. In this particular instance, the attacker has his left leg forward and is in a left forward stance; therefore his balance is weakest to his right side. And that's the area I will exploit with a propping ankle throw.

Just a quick recap: The attacker threw a right roundhouse punch, I block struck his inside forearm with my left arm. As the block strike powers into its target, I open my left hand and grasp the attacker's inside forearm and then pulled it sharply towards my left side.

Simultaneously, using my right hand, I grasp the collar of the attacker's jacket and push from my right to my left. Now both the right and left hands are working to draw the attacker off balance to his right side. The attacker now becomes unbalanced with his body weight shifting towards his toes; I move my left leg forward and use my left foot to prop against the inside of his right foot. All of this is shown in illustration 13, d. The three arrows in the same illustration will help guide you through the arms and leg movement.

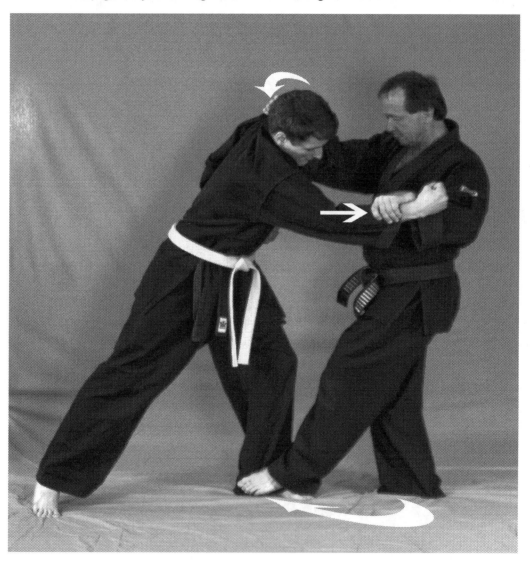

Illustration 13, d.

This throw is a classic simple throw that has been utilized in hundreds of thousands of fights since mankind has been on this earth: stick your foot out and trip your opponent up. That's exactly what I have done, but to make it more effective, I have also added the arm work that draws the attacker into the correct position to optimise the blocking/propping foot position. Hence the name, Lifting Pulling Ankle Block.

Illustration 13, e shows my left foot blocking the attacker's left foot and he is been drawn further off balance. This is the point of no return, within the next millisecond the attacker will have been thrown with some considerable force to the floor or mats. The two white arrows indicate the direction that the attacker is been drawn into to finalise the execution of the throw.

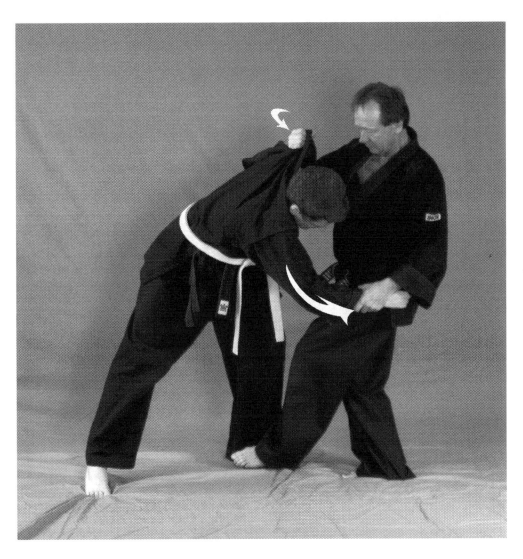

Illustration 13, e.

I am always ready for some form of retaliation from the attacker, even when a person is hurt from a heavy throw, they will still try to fight back. So as the attacker crashes into the floor, he almost lands on his left side, this makes it difficult to throw a punch with his left hand. To frustrate him further, I have kept control of his right arm by maintaining my grip of his right wrist with my left hand.

Illustration 13, f shows the attacker now on the floor/mats, suffering from the impact of the throw and me controlling his right arm, ready for any fight back.

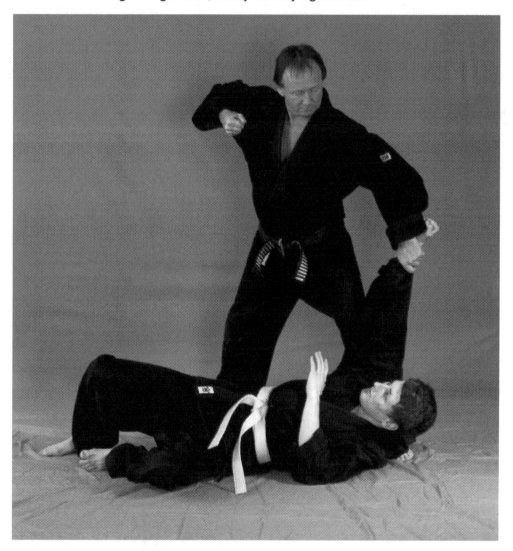

Illustration 13, f.

To finalize this routine, I drop into a deep left sided forward stance. As I do this, I extend the attacker's right arm so that his right elbow joint is resting across my left inner thigh, this starts to apply an elbow lock. To increase the pressure or indeed to break the arm at its elbow joint, I push downward with my left hand. Simultaneously, I strike the attacker's right rib area with my right fist, this will immobilise the attacker while I make my exit. If you are practicing this, kiai with the punch to the ribs for added power.

The conclusion of this routine is shown in illustration 13, g.

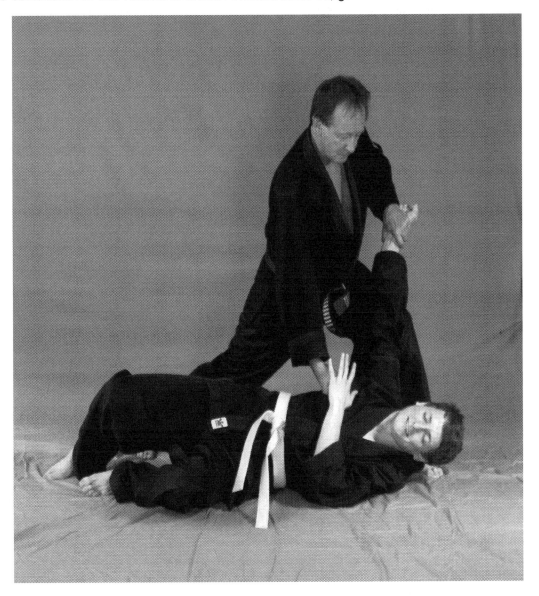

Illustration 13, g.

As always, when finishing with one attacker, just as a precaution, immediately adopt a fighting stance. You never know who may want to join in this attack! It is always better to be safe sorry.

The next few throws haven't had the historical publicity that is customary with many other classical throws. They are however age-old classics that have never really been given age old names or a categorised recognition. With this in mind, I will create a piece of Ju-Jutsu history and put a name and category to these throws: Category; Leverage throws. Types of throws; front leverage throw, back leverage throw and side leverage throw. Japanese names?

The initial throwing principle is the same as all other throws, working on getting ones opponent off balance. You then apply a fulcrum and lever principle to apply the correct leverage to throw that person. In the following pages, I will explain in detail how to execute these throws from various attacks.

Front leverage throw from the attack, both lapels held.

To kick start this routine, I have had my training partner attack me by grabbing a hold of both of my lapels. To maintain my balance, I have brought my left leg forward. This is shown in illustration 14, a.

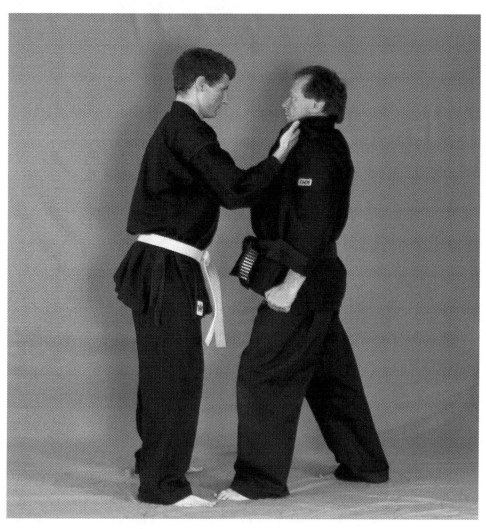

Illustration 14, a.

The attacker has tied up his two of his major weapons, his hands. I still have to be aware that he can still head butt or knee kick me. To avoid any of these, I have to move fast!

Straddle stances are often used in Ju-Jutsu to assist with defences or as part of the actual technique. For my next movement, I will drop quickly into a low straddle stance by advancing my right leg forward, placing my right foot deep in the middle of the attacker's legs. As I do this, I crash my right shoulder into the attacker's lower abdomen, this starts to unbalance him.

As a preventative measure, I drop head to the attacker's right side. This is done to avoid any head butts that could land maliciously, involuntary or accidentally.

The above movements are shown in illustration 14, b. The curved white arrow shows the direction that I have dropped my head into to avoid any head butts; the white arrow on the floor/mats shows how I advanced my right foot deep in the middle of the attacker's legs to achieve the low straddle stance.

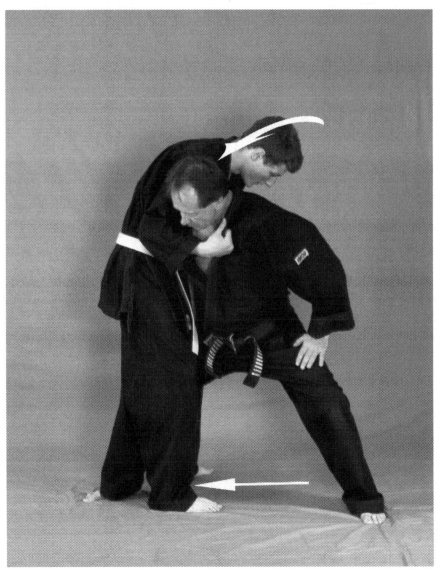

Illustration 14, b.

No attacker will ever just fall over for you. You need to constantly work on weakening any physical resistance. In this instance, I use my right open hand to strike upwards into the attacker's groin. This has an immediate effect! Even someone high on class A drugs, drunk out of there head on alcohol or been sniffing glue or other substances, will respond to a good strike to the groin!

For every action or strike that I do to the attacker, there will a reaction. From the groin strike, the attacker has reacted by bending forward. This is a natural reaction and is all part of the plan to set the attacker up ready for the throw.

Illustration 14, c shows the attacker about to be hit in the groin with my right hand.

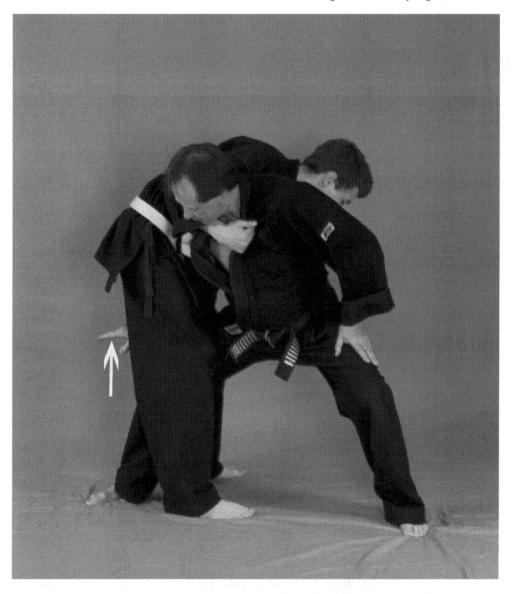

Illustration 14, c.

Note: I have used an open handed technique so that the finger's can flick strike the attacker's groin area.

As soon as the strike to the groin lands, I rapidly remove my right hand and then place my right forearm across the attacker's right upper thigh and push forward; this will act as a fulcrum. It also assists with the throw by pushing the attacker hips away from me and driving the attacker off balance. His body weight now shifts to his heels.

Illustration 14, d shows my right forearm being placed at the top of the attacker's thigh. The white arrow indicates the direction to push.

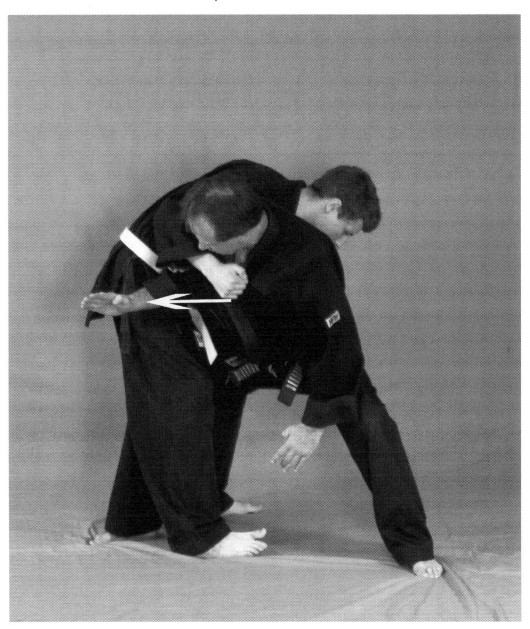

Illustration 14, d.

As I push forward with my right forearm, I reach down with my left hand and grab the back of the attacker's right ankle.

I now have the perfect fulcrum and lever, my right forearm pushes forward, to give this movement a little more weight, I also push with my right shoulder. The left hand pulls backward in an upward arc, levering the attacker's right leg up off the floor/mats. The attacker can no longer keep his balance and starts to fall backward.

Illustration 14, e shows my left hand grasping the back of the attacker's right ankle. With everything now in place, the front leverage throw can now be executed and the attacker starts to be thrown backward.

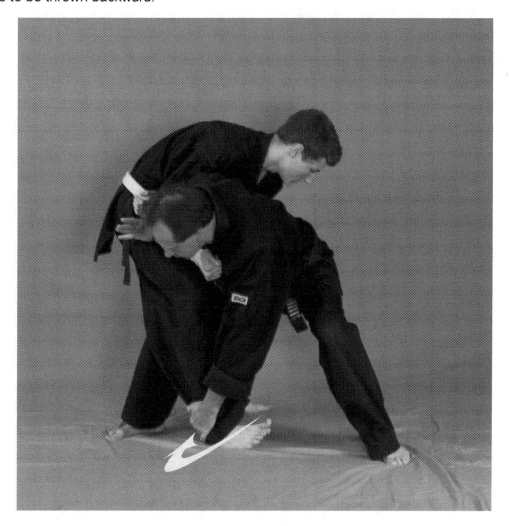

Illustration 14, e.

As the attacker falls away from me, I accelerate his descent by pulling upward sharply with my left hand. Even on mats, the impact from this throw is heavy; on a hard surface it's devastating!

Illustration 14, f shows the attacker thrown flat on his back, I am now almost standing upright after drawing the attacker's right leg upward with my right hand. The large white curved arrow indicates the path my left hand took to pull the attacker's leg upwards.

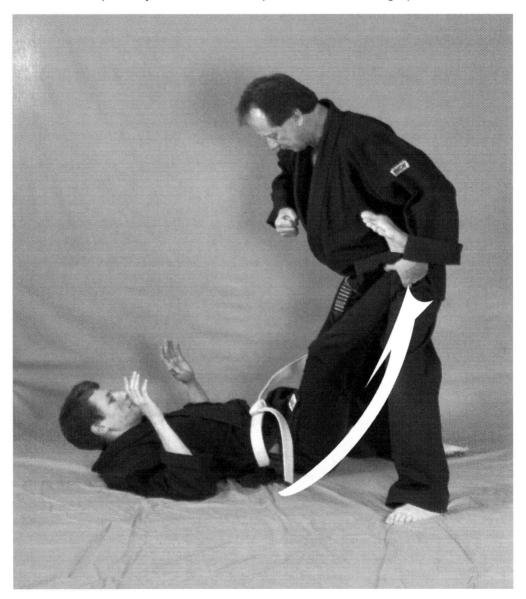

Illustration 14, f.

Please note; for safety, although my training partner has been thrown backward, he has kept his head up away from the floor/mats. This is something you must do if you practice this throw or any other throw where you fall backwards, forwards or sideways. Remember, heads, mats or floors don't mix!

To finalize this throwing routine, I keep a firm hold of the attacker's right leg with my left hand, this stops any fight back from this limb. Then in simultaneous movements, I drop down sharply with my right knee, performing a dropping knee kick into the attacker's groin and if the attacker thinks that's bad, I also punch him in the solar plexus with my right hand!

These two movements should subdue the attacker while I make a safe exit. If you are practising this, kiai with the punch and dropping knee kick for more power.

Illustration 14, g shows the attacker getting the "good news" from my right knee and right fist at the end of the front leverage throw defence routine.

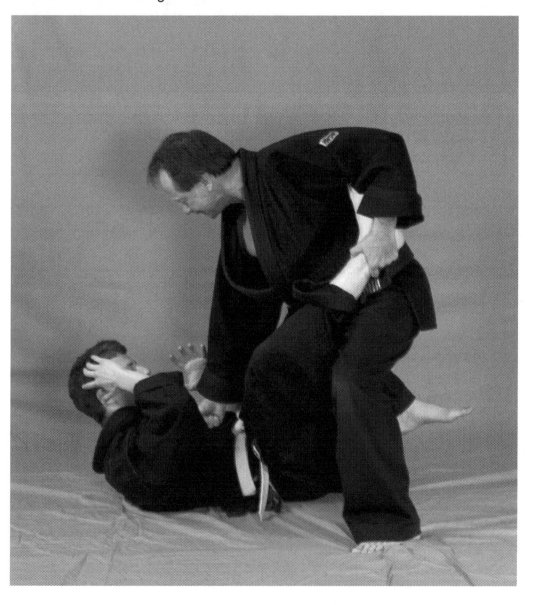

Illustration 14, g.

Just a friendly reminder, once you feel confident on one side, practise this routine on the other side.

Rear leverage throw, from a side blow to the head.

To illustrate the start of the defence routine that leads into a rear leverage throw, I and my training partner and I have come into left fighting stances, with our guards up. My training partner will once again assume the role of the attacker. His attack will be an over exaggerated side blow (big round house punch) to the side of my head. This is the kind of punch that would be thrown by someone who is drunk, drugged or just not a great fighter. It isn't the fastest punch in the world, but if you are on the receiving end, it can still make you see stars!

To do a rear leverage throw, I will have to get around to the back of the attacker; the route I have chosen for this is to duck under the attacker's side blow. Ducking under side blows takes lots of practise; you have to get your timing spot on. If you want to try this, get your training partner to throw slow side blows first. As you become more competent in ducking and slip streaming the blow, get him or her to increase the speed of the attack.

Illustration 15, a, shows me in a left fighting stance, guard up, ready for the attacker to throw a right handed side blow.

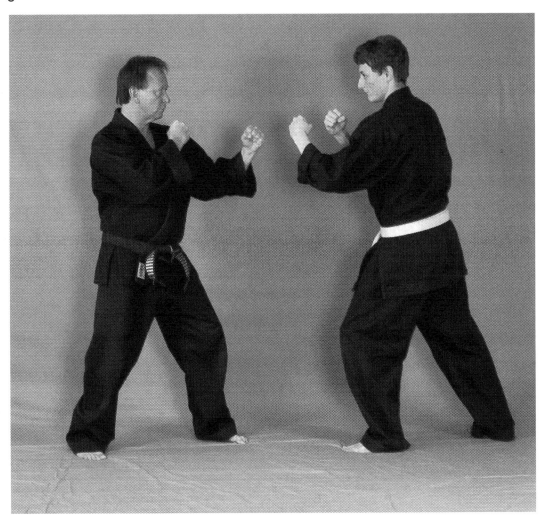

Illustration 15, a.

From his left fighting stance, the attacker steps forward with his right leg, throwing the right handed exaggerated side blow (big round house punch). To avoid the blow, I step to the attacker's right side with my left leg and drop into a low forward stance. As I step, I duck down under the attacker's striking arm, both the step and the duck are done simultaneously.

In coordination with the step and duck, I use my right hand and palm heel the attacker in the solar plexus. This strike causes him to jolt forward and is part of the initial unbalancing procedure. The palm heel is used as it aligns itself to the angle of the attacker's body. If you tried to do the same with a punch, the angle would be wrong and you could possibly injure or break your wrist!

Illustration 15, b shows the attacker been hit in the solar plexus with a palm heel strike after I ducked to his right side to avoid the side blow. The curved white arrow indicates the direction my right hand has taken to deliver the palm heel strike. The other curved arrow indicates the direction the attacker threw his side blow in.

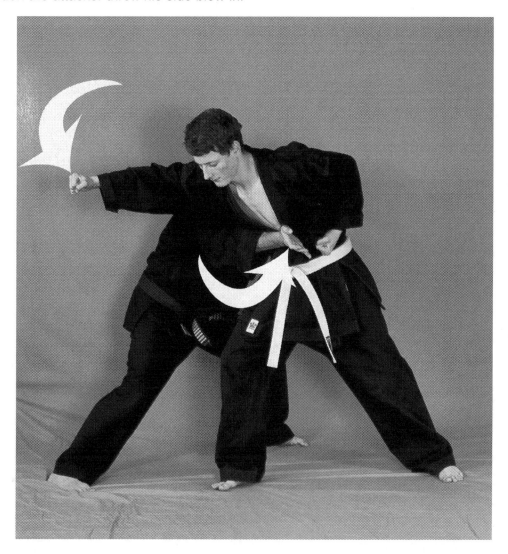

Illustration 15, b.

As the attacker reacts to the palm heel strike to the stomach, I instantly change direction with my left foot and step deep in between the attackers legs. My upper left thigh makes heavy contact with the back of the attacker's right leg nudging him forward. The actual point of contact becomes the fulcrum for this throw.

In a simultaneous movement, I reach up with my left hand, placing it on the back of the attacker's neck and then push forward; this enhances his unbalancing position by driving him forward so that his body weight shifts to his toes.

Illustration 15, c shows that my left foot has stepped deep in between the attacker's legs with a small white arrow indicating the direction I used. The curved with arrow indicates the direction my left hand has taken to push the attacker forward. The other white arrow shows that I am preparing to reach forward with my right hand and grasp the attacker's leg, just above the ankle.

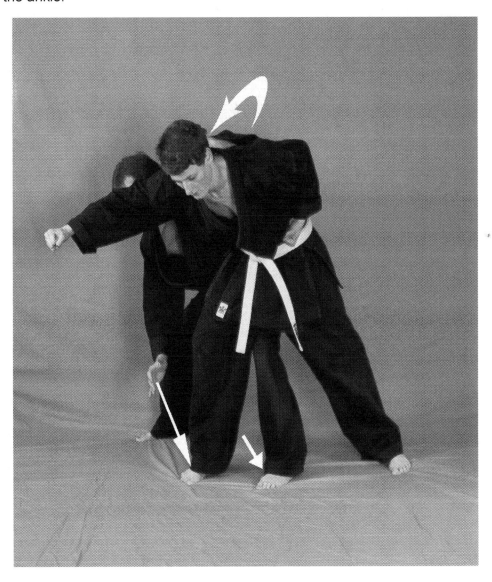

Illustration 15, c.

Using my right hand, I hook it in front of the attacker's lower right shin and start to pull backward, (this is a lever). Every thing is now in place; however this is an unusual throw as it has two levers, the lower and upper lever.

Using my left leg (fulcrum) as the central pivot point, I pull with the lower lever being my right hand and push with upper lever being my left hand. This propels the attacker forward into the throw.

Both illustrations 15,d and 15 e show the attacker falling forward at different stages with the curved arrows indicating the pull and push method for this throw.

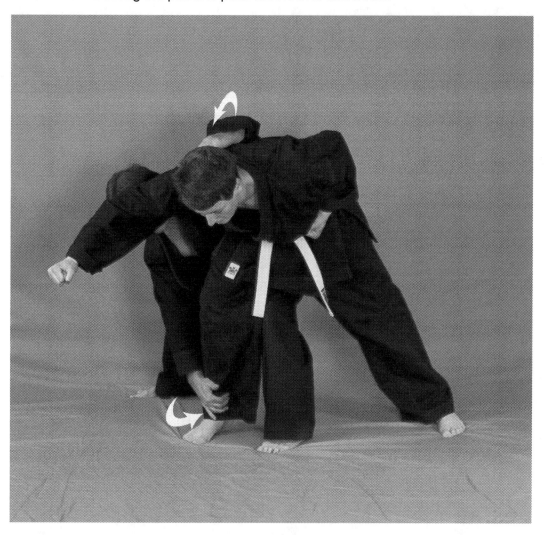

Illustration 15, d.

In illustration 15, e. the attacker is now beyond the point of no return and is been thrown face forward towards the floor, or in my case the mats.

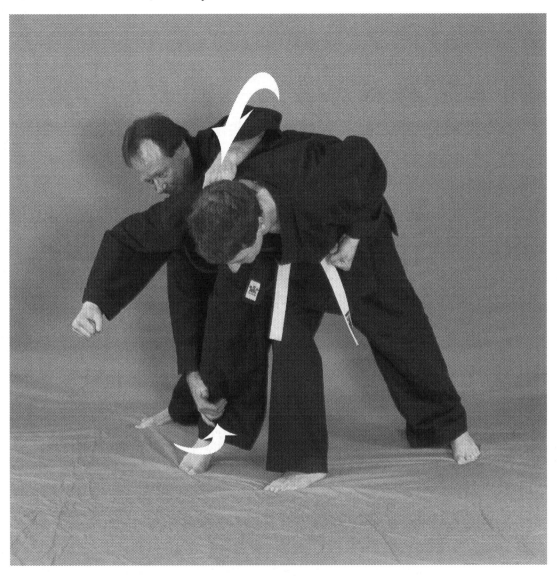

Illustration 15, e.

Once I feel I cannot push any more with my left hand, I remove it from its upper lever position and utilize it with my right hand on the lower lever. Now both my hands are holding the attacker's lower right leg and are pulling upwards. This further accelerates the rear leverage throw and the attacker falls with even more force, face first into the floor!

This would be a bad fall out in the street, most people try to save themselves from facial or head injury by putting their hands out first, but this often results in both wrists been badly injured or broken!

Caution! When you practice this, make sure your training partner knows how to do a front breakfall.

Illustration 15, f shows the attacker face down on the floor/mats and me pulling upward with both of my hands. The white arrow in this illustration is self explanatory.

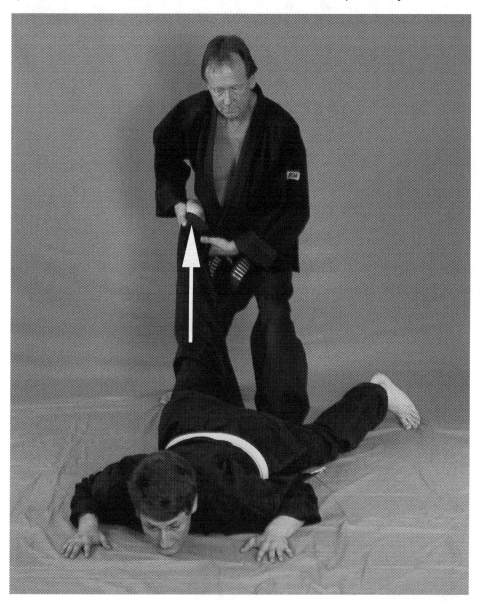

Illustration 15, f.

To conclude this throwing routine, I have kept a hold of the attacker's right leg with my right hand and pull upwards; this raises the attacker's right hip off the floor. With his leg and hip elevated, It naturally exposes the attacker's groin area to a kick that can only be described as a "mans nightmare." I will leave you to imagine what this might entail.

Illustration 15, g shows the completion of the rear leverage throw, from a side blow to the head with the attacker getting an unusual, but effective kick in the groin.

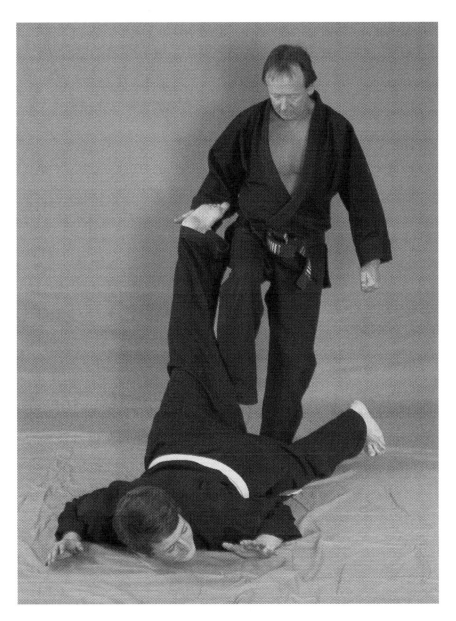

Illustration 15, g.

If this were a real defence routine out in the street, I would disengage the attacker's leg and assume a fighting stance in anticipation of any other potential attacker's.

Remember, if you try this routine, practice the throw right and left.

Aiki throwing techniques

The next range of throwing techniques are Aiki variants that come under the term Aiki-jūjutsu. Aiki-jūjutsu is a form of jujutsu which emphasizes "an early neutralization of an attack. **They are definitely not pure Aikido** (合気道 *aikidō*).

The exact origins of these individual throwing techniques have been lost in ancient times; however styles such as **Daitō-ryū Aiki-jūjutsu** (大東流合気柔術) encapsulated the purer form of these throwing techniques into their ryu (school) and they themselves maintain a linage with the Shinra Saburō Minamoto no Yoshimitsu (新羅 三郎 源 義光, 1045–1127), who was a Minamoto clan samurai and member of the Seiwa Genji (the branch of the Minamoto family descending from 56th imperial ruler of Japan, Emperor Seiwa). I make no claim or link to the above.

The word "aikido" is formed of three kanji:

合 - *ai* - joining, harmonizing

気 - *ki* - spirit, life energy.

道 - *dō* - way, path. The term dō connects the practice of aikido with the philosophical concept of *Tao*, which can be found in martial arts such as judo and kendo, and in more peaceful arts such as Japanese calligraphy (shodō), flower arranging (kadō) and tea ceremony (chadō or sadō).

Aiki is a Japanese martial arts principle or tactic. In Japanese Aiki is formed from two kanji: 合 - ai - joining, harmonizing, 気 - ki - spirit, life energy.

Jutsu (術?) — meaning technique, method, skill or trick — is a bound morpheme of the Sino-Japanese lexical stratum of the Japanese language. Jutsu may combine with another morpheme (or word) to form a word. It does so much more commonly as a second part; examples are, jūjutsu (柔術, unarmed fighting) battōjutsu (抜刀術, the art of drawing a sword)

Jujutsu (柔術 *jūjutsu*) literally meaning the "art of softness", or "way of yielding" is a collective name for Japanese martial art styles consisting of grappling and striking techniques.

When one looks at the history of Aikido as a pure art, it derived its core techniques from **Daitō-ryū** and certain modern day Ryu's (Schools) have claimed exclusivity of these techniques. While some controversy exists and will always exist as to the ownership of these throwing techniques, they are indeed an intricate part of many ancient and modern Ju-Jutsu systems including my own.

Thoughts on Aiki.

The oldest book to discuss aiki was the 1899 Budo Hiketsu-Aiki no Jutsu. On the subject of aiki it was written:

The most profound and mysterious art in the world is the art of aiki. This is the secret principle of all the martial arts in Japan. One who masters it can be an unparalleled martial genius.

The Textbook of Jujutsu (Jujutsu Kyoju-sho Ryu no Maki) from 1913 wrote:

Aiki is an impassive state of mind without a blind side, slackness, evil intention, or fear. There is no difference between aiki and ki-ai; however, if compared, when expressed dynamically aiki is called kiai, and when expressed statically, it is aiki.

Aiki-jūjutsu, the Principle of Circular Motion

Aiki and Aiki-jūjutsu are unique in that they use total body movements to create a spherical motion around a stable, energized centre. Regardless of the ways the opponent attacks, through precise usage of leverage, inertia, gravity, and the action of centrifugal and centripetal forces, the opponent will be easily overcome and thrown. Ultimately, it is the energy of the attack itself which brings down the attacker.

Evasive body movement, TAI SABAKI 体捌き.

All Aikido, Aiki-jutsu and Aiki-jujutsu styles have the same unique evasive foot work or body turning movement; this is called TAI SABAKI 体捌き. Tai sabaki is usually used to avoid an attack, in certain techniques it is used in conjunction with other body movements and it is this combination that makes the technique flow. This implies the use of harmonization rather than physical strength.

The concept of Aiki jūjutsu

1) Blending not clashing. 2) Dominating the assailant. 3) Use of internal strength - Ki energy

Go with the flow

To try to make life easier, I have my own term that fits Aiki-ju-jutsu based techniques that I teach, "going with the flow".

The idea of "going with the flow" sounds easy, but it is one of the most difficult things to learn. Why? Because we all initially have a natural tendency to try to utilise our own physical strength to defeat our attacker's.

Aiki techniques are unique in that you learn to blend in with the attacker's movements and through the applied technique, you control the attacker to the point where you can throw him or her with minimal effort. This does not mean that the attacker gets of lightly! Each throwing technique is extremely powerful and the final "ground hitting impact" is as hard as any Judo throw I know.......In some cases harder!!!

To understand the "go with the flow principle" I have linked a sequence of photographs together so that you can see how I have blended in with the attacker's momentum. To capture the action, I have used a high speed digital SLR camera that records at 5 shots per second. My (Uke 受け the person who will initiate an attack against the thrower) will be attacking me at full speed.

The perfect attack!

This seems like a good time to mention "the perfect attack". Not all, but many modern day martial arts train the (Uke) attacker to do a stylised attack that conforms to the ideology of their particular style. While this has certain visual values that make both the attack and defence pleasing to the eye and also makes the art or style look good, it has no value in the real world where the attacker will just simply attack you! So let's put attacks into their correct prospective. Real attacks by their nature are both violent, crude, they have no style and there is **no wrong way** for the attacker or attacker's to come at you. To sum up, **there is no perfect attack**, you just have to accept the attack, go with the flow and apply the appropriate defence.

While I was writing this last paragraph, I came across a video clip on YouTube that highlights "the perfect attack" and its pitfalls. The clip is a comedy sketch done by the American comedian Jim Carey; in it he plays the part of a martial arts teacher. If you get a chance have a look at it, you will then see what I am ranting on about, this is the YouTube link; http://uk.youtube.com/watch?v=h_vvl26NnwE. Enjoy it.

Four-direction throw.

The first throw in this range I would like to show you is a **Four-direction throw or four corner throw** (四方投げ *shihōnage*).

This throwing technique is done where the defender passes under attacker's arm, then lifts it overhead, pivots 180 degrees and throws.

1. The routine starts with both of use in a fighting stance; I have my left leg forward.

2. The attacker lunges forward with a right handed downward blow, I immediately prepare to blend in with the attack by dropping both my arms at about a forty five degree angle to my right side.

3. As the attacker's right arm starts to descend, I raise my left arm up ready to parry the blow.

4. I start to move forward with my right leg and use my left open hand to blend in with the attacker's blow.

5. Having completed my step forward (Tai sabaki) with my right leg, in a circular motion I start to feed the attacker's arm from my left to my right hand.

6. With the attacker's right hand secured with my left and right hands, I continue to draw his arm from his right to his left side.

7. Continuing the circular motion, I raise the attacker's right arm upward and start to step forward with my left leg, this starts to break the attacker's balance.

8. With both arms raised up high, I complete the step forward with my left leg and then immediately pivot 180 degrees on both feet and change direction.

9. Keeping the circular motion going, the attacker's right hand is folded back past the shoulder, locking the shoulder joint. I then start to step forward with my right leg; this now has the attacker off balance**.**

Illustration 16, a, pictures 1 to 9.

Four-direction throw (四方投げ *shihōnage*)

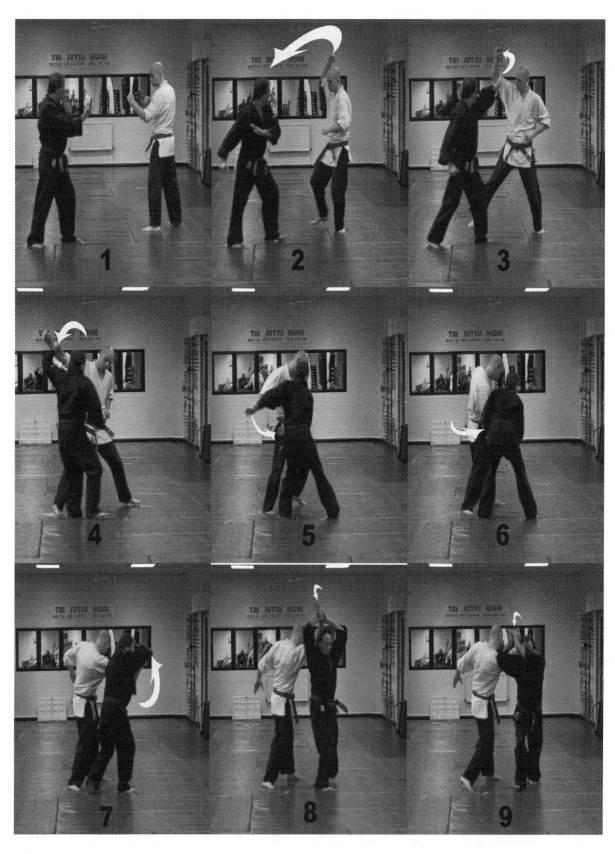

10. I continue to step with my right foot and draw the attacker further off balance.

11. To compensate for the attacker being taller than I am and to enhance the unbalancing of the attacker, I begin to take another step with my left leg.

12. The attacker is thrown to the mats/floor.

13. The technique is completed with me keeping the flow going by extending both my arms forward and ending up in left forward stance.

Illustration 16, b, pictures 10 to 13. **Four-direction throw** *(四方投げ shihōnage)*

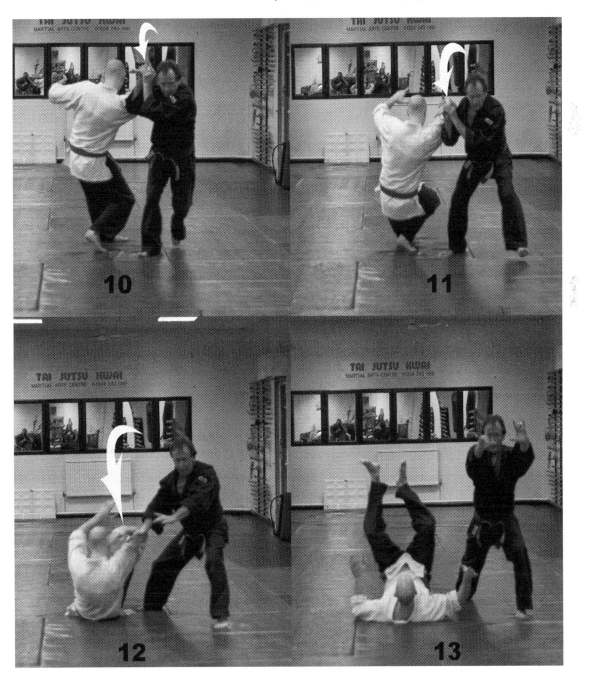

If you have a go a this technique, take it slow at first, break it down into the 1 to 13 stages and then as you get the idea and you feel the technique starting to flow, increase your speed. Once you really feel confident, try it on the opposite side.

Warning: Don't bang the shoulder lock on as shown in pictures 8 through to 12 or you will dislocate your training partners shoulder!

Heaven-and-earth throw

Heaven-and-earth throw (天地投げ *tenchinage)*. A technique where one brings one's hand/forearm upward (heaven) under the chin of the attacker and then downward with the other hand (earth) to execute the throw.

This is the next technique to have a look at. I have chosen this one because it epitomizes what aiki based techniques are about; minimal effort, maximum results and that all important flow.

Safety

Before you try this throw make sure your training partner knows how the breakfall correctly as the heaven-and-earth throw is known in the martial arts world as one of the most powerful and fastest throwing techniques. When your training partner hits the mats, he or she will be travelling at a fair old MPH. Also look at the final picture number 9, you can see that my training partner's head is well away from the mats, remember...........heads and mats don't mix!

I have seen a few nasty accidents that could have been easily avoided. So another safety hint is; make sure you warn your training partner to close their mouth and keep their tongue well away from his or her teeth when you raise your arm upward in pictures 4,5,6,7 of illustration 17, a.

1. The action starts for the heaven and earth throw with both I and the attacker have coming into a fighting stance with our left legs forward.

2. As the attacker instigates the attack, a lunge punch with his right fist. I move my left hand in the start of a circle to my left side.

3. I quarter step with my left foot so that my body is out of line from the attacker's punch. At the same time, I continue the circular motion with my left hand so it now raised up above the attacker's striking arm.

4. My left arm drops down on the top of the attacker's right attacking arm, at the same time I swing my right arm to my right side, this allows my body to flow naturally and sets the right arm up for the next movement.

5. Using my left hand, I continue the circular motion and draw the attacker's right arm down away from his right side. Keeping the flow going, I raise my right arm upward and make contact with my forearm just under the attack's chin. This is the classic heaven and earth arm position.

6. I begin the step forward with my right leg and at the same time I raise both arms up and start to push forward, this starts to drive the attacker off balance.

7. I continue to step forward with my right leg and drive the attacker further off balance.

8. The attacker is partially thrown to the floor; however I keep the flow of power going.

9. The technique is completed with me ending up in a strong right sided forward stance, both arms extended forward and the attacker hitting the floor/mats with extreme force.

Illustration 17, a pictures 1 to 9, **Heaven-and-earth throw** *(天地投げ tenchinage)*

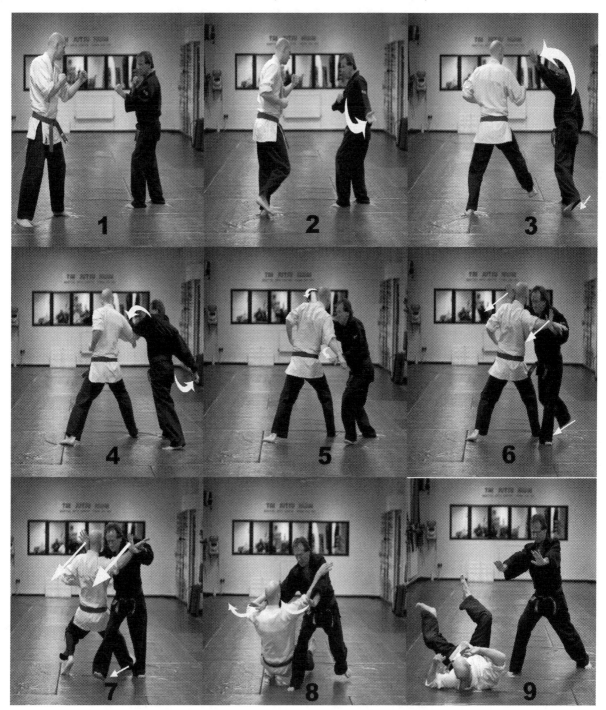

For the Street Only

To add some more clout into this throw, a couple of small but devastating variations can be done from "a street point of view only". In illustration 17, a, pictures 4, 5, 6, use your forearm to strike or in wrestling terms "clothesline" the attacker across the throat. Or instead of clothes lining the attacker use pictures 4, 5, 6 and change them for an uppercut. This will launch any attacker into space!!!

Finally, attacker's throw punches with lefts as well as rights, so once you have practiced this throwing technique on the one side, remember to give it a go on the other side.

Entering throw or Enter Body throw

Entering throw or Enter Body throw (入身投げ *iriminage*). The classic form superficially resembles a "clothesline" technique. Irimi means, entering (movement); direct inward movement by the defender in front or to the rear of the attacker prior to the execution of a technique. Nage means, throw or projection.

Note; to help you understand this technique and to follow the enter body throw routine more clearly; I have superimposed a knife into the attacker's hand. From a street point of view, I personally would only use this technique against a blunt weapon.

Safety

To keep your training partner safe and from having his or her teeth knocked out! Make sure there mouths are closed, tongue away from the teeth, especially when you get to picture 8!

1. The attacker has squared up to me, left leg forward and has a knife (superimposed) in his right hand. I have immediately come into a right sided knife fighting stance.

2. The attackers raise's the knife above his head and begins to step forward with his right leg. I prepare to blend in with the attack by lowering both arms below my belt line.

3. The attacker now steps further forward. I begin to raise both hands upward in an arc.

4. As the attacker starts to slash downward, I raise both arms up further. My right hand is now in position to be able to parry the attacker's knife hand. At the same time, I begin to move forward with my left leg (Tai sabaki), this moves my body out of the attacker's "cutting" line.

5. My right hand has parried the attacker's right knife hand downward; at the same time my left hand has now been placed on the side of the attacker's neck.

6. Using both my right and left hands, I draw the attacker forward so that his body weight shifts to his front foot; this slows the attacks momentum down.

7. I then pivot my body 180 degrees and step away from the attacker with my left leg. At the same time, I begin to raise my right arm upward.

8. My right forearm makes contact under the attacker's chin in the classic "clothesline." This starts to drive the attacker off balance. In the same motion, I move my left hand from the attacker's neck and place it on his right shoulder and push inward, this enhances the unbalancing action.

9. As the attacker becomes more off balance, I start to drive my right arm downward. At the same time I begin to step forward with my right leg.

Illustration 18, a, pictures 1 to 9. **Entering throw or Enter Body throw** *(入身投げ iriminage)*

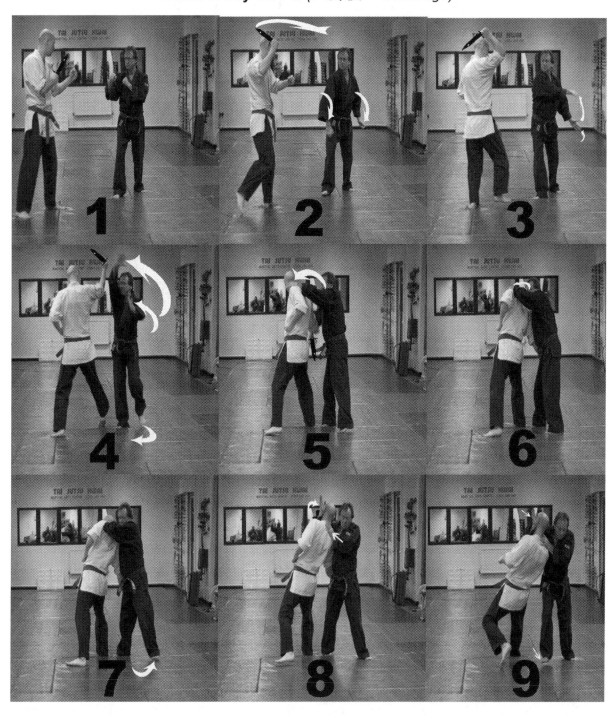

10. I complete my step forward with my right leg and continue to drive the attacker to the floor/mats.

11. As I feel the attacker accelerate away from me, I extend both my arms down at about a forty five degree angle. This keeps the flow on power going and adds more force to the throw.

12. As the attacker impacts on the floor, I begin to raise my arm up to about my shoulder height.

13. The technique is completed with me stabilising my posture and I end up in a right sided forward stance. My both arms are extended forward to complete the flow of power.

Illustration 18, b, pictures 10 to 13. Entering throw or Enter Body throw
(入身投げ iriminage)

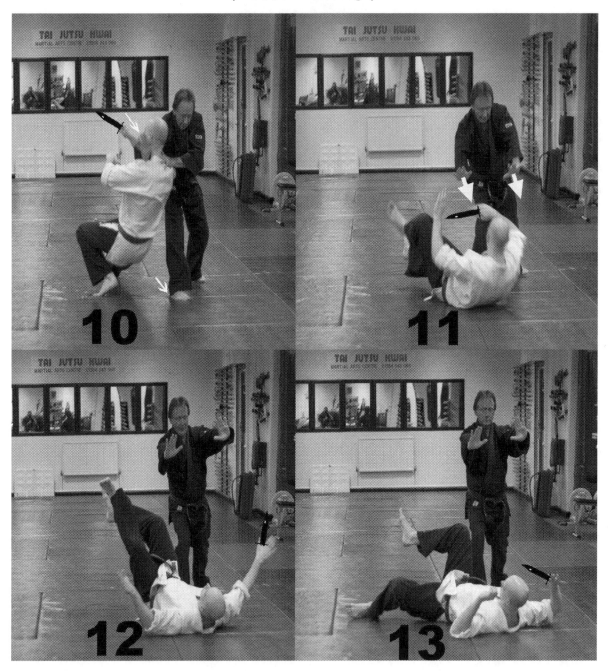

Once you try one side switch over and give the other side a go. I know I am repeating myself, but that's what martial arts have done for me, it has made me extremely methodical.

This also concludes the basic throwing section of this book, I hope the techniques described give you a better understanding of the immense variety of throws there are in Ju-Jutsu and how throws work.

Stranglehold or chokehold techniques

When you have been on Ju-Jutsu classes for a little while, it is highly probable that you will be taught a stranglehold or chokehold technique. These come under the title of *shime-waza*, 絞技, " shime" means constriction, "waza" means technique.

Let's talk about Safety first.

As these techniques are extremely dangerous in that they can render the recipient unconscious or indeed dead, all Ju-Jutsu clubs have safety practice procedures that must be observed. The Instructor or Sensei should methodically go through these safety procedures prior to and when practicing these highly dangerous technique.

If however you have never been to a Ju-Jutsu class, the basic rules are as follows;

Rule 1. Strangulation and Choking techniques must be taught and supervised by a qualified instructor. Qualified instructor means the Sensei, not one of class students or assistants.

Rule 2. A qualified first aider or qualified Sensei who is familiar with Katsu or Kappo (Resuscitation Techniques) should always be present. Note: Although a person has a first aid certificate, it does not necessarily mean they are competent to resuscitate a person who has who has become unconscious from a strangulation technique (shime-waza).

Rule 3. When applying a strangulation or choking technique, you must release pressure immediately when the opponent submits. This is indicated by the recipient tapping his opponent or the mat twice; however common sense should prevail, if the person starts going limp, blue or coughing, then stop immediately!

Rule 4. Extra care should be taken when applying strangulation or choking technique to those who are weaker than you. This will effectively apply to women and children whose physiology is different to adult males.

Rule 5. Do not take unnecessary risks; learn to give in when a technique is being applied to you.

Rule 6. You never practice or show any of the Strangulation and Choking techniques outside the Dojo (martial arts place of leaning). If you do you can expect to be expelled from your martial arts club.

What are Strangulation and Choking techniques?

They are methods of applying compression to the neck that results in choking, unconsciousness or death by causing an increasingly hypoxic state in the brain.

Definition of **hypoxia:** Hypoxia generally refers to a lack of oxygen in any part of the body. In a neurological context, it refers to a reduction of oxygen to the brain despite adequate amounts of blood

In martial arts terms these methods are all classed under one term *shime-waza*, 絞技," shime means constriction, waza means technique". But in plain English, a Choke and a Strangle are classified as two different things.

Why are they classed as the same?

The answer to this is simple, when you apply a martial arts Shime-waza, you often, through the nature of the technique, apply both choke and strangle techniques at the same time.

To analyse the effects of strangulation and choking techniques individually, the results are as follows;

Strangulation techniques

<u>Shime-waza,</u> Strangulation techniques involves one or several mechanisms that interfere with the normal flow of oxygen into the brain: Depending on how the strangling is performed, it may compress the airway, interfere with the flow of blood in the neck, or work as a combination of the two. Often compression through strangulation techniques of the carotid arteries or jugular vein causes cerebral ischemia. Compression of the laryngopharynx, larynx or trachea causes asphyxia. Complete obstruction of blood flow to the brain is associated with irreversible neurological damage and death. A well applied strangulation technique to the larynx or trachea is almost instantaneous, in practice, your training partner will be submitting immediately.

Definitions

Jugular veins: Veins which return blood from the head and neck to the heart.

Carotid arteries: The left and right common carotid arteries are the principal arteries supplying the head and neck. Each has two main branches, external carotid artery and internal carotid artery.

Larynx: valve structure between the trachea (windpipe) and the pharynx (the upper throat) that is the primary organ of voice production.

Trachea: A thin-walled, cartilaginous tube descending from the larynx to the bronchi and carrying air to the lungs. Also called a windpipe.

Asphyxia: Interference with circulation and oxygenation of the blood that leads to loss of consciousness and possible brain damage.

Cerebral ischemia: Global Brain Ischemia is when blood ceases to flow or the blood flow to the brain decreases drastically.

Choke techniques

Shime-waza, choke or carotid restraint specifically refers to a chokehold or a blood choke that compresses one or both carotid arteries and/or the jugular veins without compressing the airway, hence causing cerebral ischemia and a temporary hypoxic condition in the brain. Regardless of whom the opponent is, a well applied choke technique leads to unconsciousness in 4-10 seconds, an expert will do it in less! After release, the subject regains consciousness spontaneously in 10-20 seconds. If this technique was applied for longer, say 30 seconds, it could result in death!

These choke holds also have the name "Sleeper hold", they are often seen in modern day wrestling bouts where the recipient appears to have gone to sleep through the application of the "sleeper hold".

When you combine the technique of strangulation and the choking together, you end up with an extremely lethal cocktail! The Shime-waza.

How safe are these techniques?

In researching strangulation techniques for this book, I found that to date their have been fourteen fatalities in applying a strangle or choke hold, thirteen of these were done by law enforcement officers and one by a student learning Vo et Vat, a Vietnamese version of judo. Looking at the case history of those thirteen fatalities from the law enforcement officers, death in most cases could have been avoided, if the person being restrained had not struggled.

Law enforcement agencies around the world have now updated their stranglehold procedures, some have abandoned strangle holds and neck restraints completely.

Those who train within martial arts have proven that over many, many years with the correct safety procedure in place, these techniques can be practiced safely. Our friends from the Japanese Sport Judo world are a shinning example of this; hundreds of thousands of these techniques have been applied in Judo competitions with no fatalities and that goes back to 1882 when Judo was started.

On a cautionary note; you must also realise that if you applied a Shime-waza in defence of your life, the attacker does not know the martial arts rules of submission. He or she will ultimately try to resist and that could be fatal for them. So my advice is, apply the Shime-waza, strangulation technique as part of your defence to stun the person and immediately switch to another technique to finalise the defence.

Hadaka jime or naked neck lock.

The first **Shime-waza,** strangulation technique that I want to show you is the classic, **Hadaka jime** or naked neck lock; this technique is applied from the rear with the forearm across the throat. I will also add an extra choke technique towards the end of this routine.

The reference to "naked" does not infer that this technique is done without any clothes on, (sorry to burst your bubble). It refers to using ones hands to apply the technique as apposed to using the attacker's clothing or if practicing, your partners Gi (martial arts suit).

To put the **Hadaka jime** technique into a Ju-Jutsu self defence routine, I have got my training partner to arm himself with a cosh; he is holding this above his head in his right hand with his left leg forward. The attack he will do is a downward blow to the head. For the rest of this routine, I will refer to him as the attacker. To ready myself for the defence, I have come into a right sided fighting stance. This is shown in illustration 19, a.

Illustration 19, a. shows the start of downward blow routine, using **Hadaka jime** *or naked neck lock as the defence.*

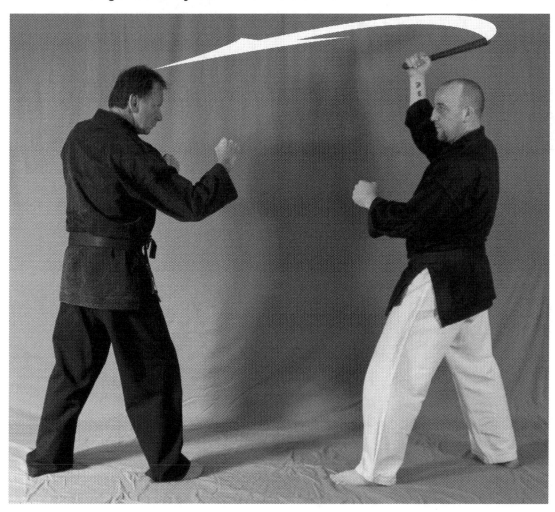

The white arrow in the above illustration shows the direction that the downward blow attack will come in from.

The attacker steps forward with his right leg and using the weapon in his right hand, he tries to strike my head with it.

As the weapon starts to descend, I raise both hands up and with open hands; I begin to parry the weapon away from its intended target………My Head!

Illustration 19, b shows the attacker's right arm being intercepted by my doubled handed parry. The two curved white arrows in this illustration show the direction my hands are moving in.

Illustration 19, b. Start of the two handed parry.

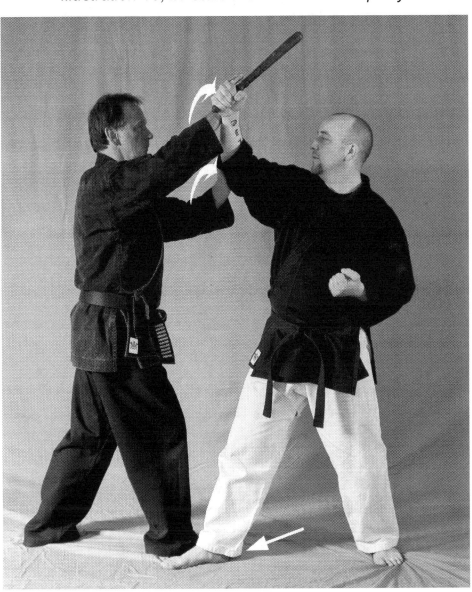

Still keeping my right leg forward, I switch from a fighting stance into a forward stance. At the same time, using both hands, I drive the attacker's right arm downward and well away from me. Note: - I am not catching his arm but guiding it away. By driving the attacker's right arm downward, it shifts his body weight heavily into his right foot. This action throws his body balance forward and momentarily slows down any possibility of a counter attack. This consequentially gives me time while I line myself up for the next part of this defence routine.

These movements are shown in illustration 19, c. The two white curved arrows in this illustration will help guide you through the parrying action I have used.

Illustration 19, c. Parrying the attackers arm.

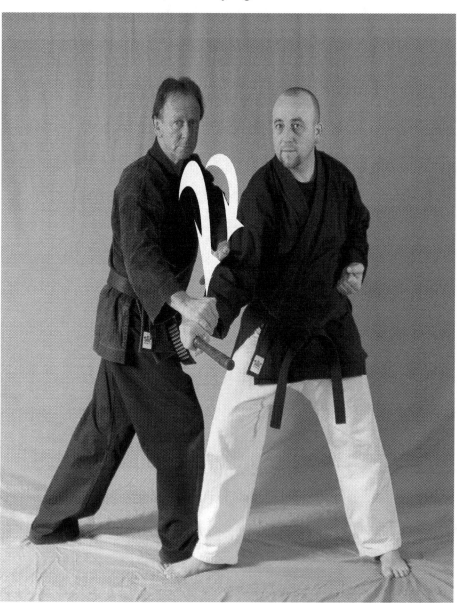

The next few movements are all done simultaneously and with a explosion of extra high-speed.

I make a small step with my right leg and a large step with my left leg to the rear of the attacker, this helps align my body for the forthcoming strangulation technique. As I do this, I remove my right hand from its parrying position, then using my right forearm I strike the attacker hard across the throat, palm facing down. The palm facing down is important as it helps set up the strangulation technique.

Illustration 19, d shows the attacker being struck across the throat with my right forearm; the curved white arrow shows its striking direction. The two straight white arrows on the floor indicate the directions I stepped with my feet.

Illustration 19, d. Striking the attacker in the throat.

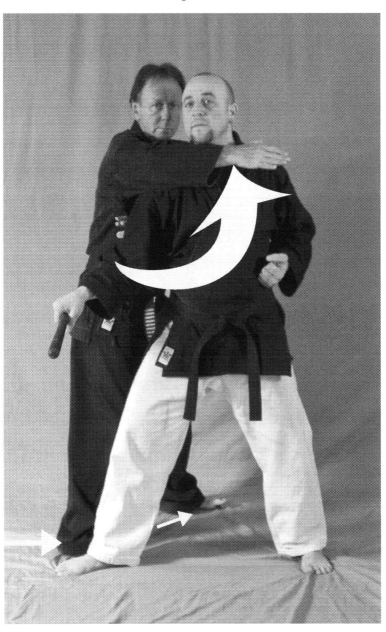

To complete my manoeuvre to the rear of the attacker, I reverse the left leg backwards; this now puts me in a strong forward stance with my right leg forward. The stance is critical, as it give stability to the strangulation technique. The manoeuvre has also aligned my head to the left of the attacker's head, this alleviates any thoughts of the attacker from trying to head butt backwards and further sets the attacker up for the imminent strangle.

In coordinated movements, using my left hand, I reach up and clasp hands together, my left hand faces upward and my right hand faces downward. I then pull backwards with both hands, drawing the attacker's head onto my right shoulder. This results in the edge of my forearm compressing the airway and strangling the attacker. This is shown in illustration 19, e. I have also added a small photo in the corner of this illustration too emphasise the hand positions in the strangulation technique.

*Illustration 19, e. The **Hadaka jime** or naked neck lock is being applied.*

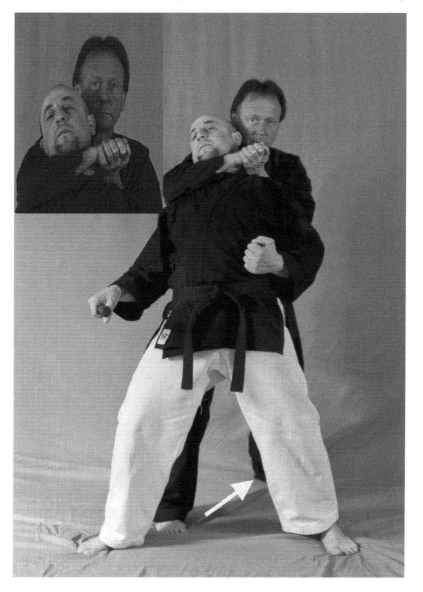

With the attacker stunned from the **Hadaka jime** or naked neck lock, I withdraw my left hand from the palm to palm position and place it on the attacker's temple area. I then push the attacker's head to his left shoulder, this now changes the strangulation into a choke and both the carotid artery and jugular vein are compressed. This is shown in illustration 19, f. The white curved arrow in this illustration indicates the direction of the push with my left hand.

Illustration 19, f. The attacker's head is pushed towards his left shoulder and a choke being applied.

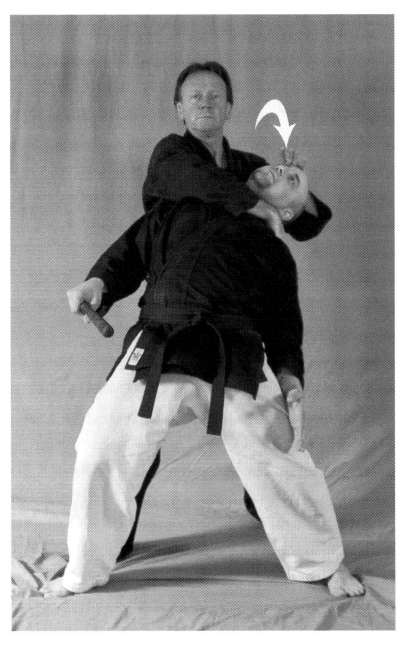

Warning: Do not apply this choke for more than a few seconds!

To conclude this routine, I pivot sharply to my left; this brings me into a left forward stance. I then raise my right arm upward and using my right elbow, I strike downward onto the attacker's right collar bone. This action can possibly break the collar bone; furthermore, a broken collar bone is the second most painful bone to break in the body (the coccyx being the first). This now should subdue the attacker long enough for me to make a speedy and safe exit.

Illustration 19, g shows the conclusion of **Hadaka jime** or naked neck lock, choke routine with an elbow strike. The white arrow shows the direction of the elbow strike.

Illustration 19, g.

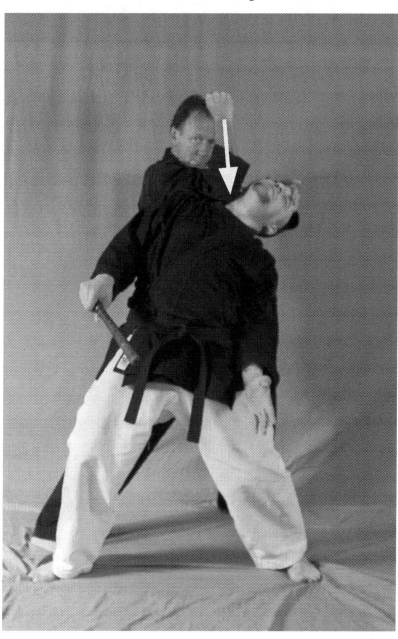

If I were dealing with this attack out in the street, I would retrieve the weapon before I exited and place it somewhere safe.

As with all the defence routines in this book, I show one side only. But, for you to learn how to defend yourself out in the street, you need to practice both sides. So once you feel you are good on one side, have a go on the other side.

Hadaka jime (naked neck lock) variation.

The next **Shime-waza** (strangulation technique), I want to show you is a powerful variation on **Hadaka jime** (naked neck lock). You could say this is its "big brother".

To set the stage for this, I and my training partner have come into fighting stances. I am leading with my right; he is leading with his left. This is shown in illustration 20, a. Note: For the rest of this routine, I shall refer to my training partner as the attacker.

Illustration 20, a. This is the start of **Hadaka jime** *(naked neck lock) variation.*

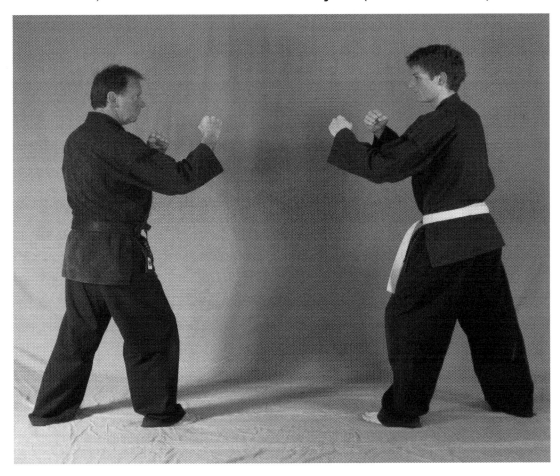

From the attacker's left fighting stance, he steps forward with his right foot and attempts to do a lunge punch (straight punch) to my face.

As part of my evasion of this attack, using my left leg, I quarter step to my immediate left. At the same time, I ward off the attacker's punching right arm with a double open handed parry. The double handed parry not only redirects the punch away from my face, it drives the attacker's arm downward and this throws his body weight into his front right foot. This tactic results in the attacker momentarily being disadvantaged and I intend to fully capitalise on this.

These movements are shown in Illustration 20, b. The two curved arrows show the direction of the doubled handed parry, while the other two straight arrow shows how the attacker has stepped and the direction of his intended punch.

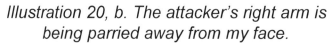

Illustration 20, b. The attacker's right arm is being parried away from my face.

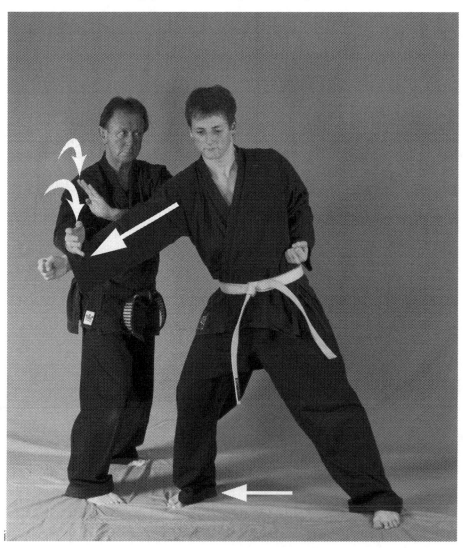

To align myself correctly, using my left foot, I step into a forward stance to the rear of the attacker. The white arrow in illustration 20, c shows the direction I stepped into and the same illustration shows my body position in relation to the attacker.

As I step to the rear of the attacker, I simultaneously strike upwards using my right forearm hitting the attacker under the chin. This strike has the same effect as an upper cut, so now the attacker's head is driven backward, this exposes the throat area ready for the strangulation technique.

The forearm strike is also shown in illustration 20, c. Its striking direction is shown by the large white curved arrow. Note: My head is to the left side of the attacker's head; this is to avoid a head collision as the attacker's head moves backward from the forearm strike.

Illustration 20, c. The attacker is struck under the chin with a forearm strike.

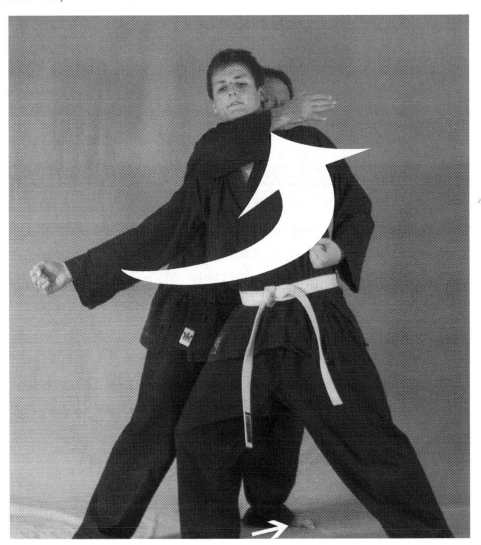

As with all the techniques that I show in this book, lots of little things happen simultaneously in each illustration I show. All of these little things are critical to the overall success of the defence routine and the execution of the named technique. This next illustration is no exception.

From my rear forward stance, I pivot forty five degrees to my right; that puts me facing the same direction as the attacker. At the same, I correct my posture by stepping back with my left leg; this posture correction puts me into a strong forward stance that is needed to support the attacker's body weight when applying the strangle hold. This is shown in illustration 20, d, the small arrow pointing to my left foot indicates my posture correction.

In simultaneous movements, I reach up high with my left arm and then using my right hand, I grasp a hold of my left bicep. These two actions are shown in illustration 20, d with arrows to help guide you through the individual movements.

Ilustration 20, d. The left arm is raised up and the right hand grasps a hold of the left bicep.

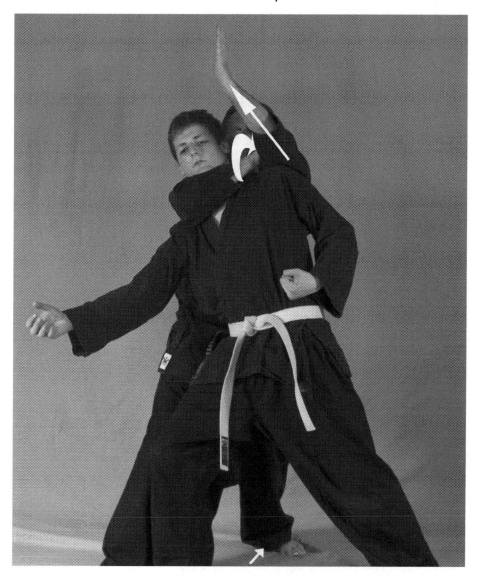

As soon as I grasp hold of my left bicep, I fold my left arm to the rear of the attacker's head. At the same time, I place my left palm on the crown area of the attacker's head. This is shown in illustration 20, e. The curved white arrow indicates the folding of my left arm. Every thing is now in place to apply the strangle hold.

In two simultaneous movements, I push forward with my left palm and draw backwards with my right forearm, this results in the trachea and larynx being simultaneously compressed. The strangulation technique is instantaneous due to the intricate leverages being applied from both arms and hands. This powerful **Shime-waza** is definitely **Hadaka jime** big brother!

Illustration 20, e shows the **Hadaka jime** (naked neck lock) variation being applied, I have also added two other small illustrations in the left and right top corners that show slightly different angles.

Illustration 20, e. **Hadaka jime** *(naked neck lock) variation being applied.*

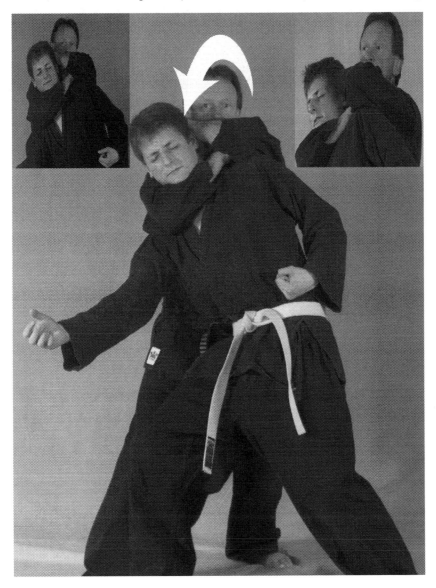

Warning: Do not "bang" this strangle hold on your training partner; it will injure him or her!

With the attacker stunned from the **Hadaka jime** (naked neck lock) variation, my right hand releases its grip of my left bicep and I then place it on the attacker's left shoulder, (this still gives me an forearm bar across the attacker's throat). Simultaneously, I slide my left hand from the crown of the attacker's head to the top of his head. These two actions only take about a millisecond to do but, in that time, I have been able to switch from the strangulation to a naked choke hold!

The naked choke hold is now simply applied by pushing my left hand sharply to my right, this drive the attacker's head sideways. This results in, extreme pressure being applied to the right side of the attacker's neck that compress's his carotid artery and jugular vein. Remember, he is also still feeling the effects of the frontal arm bar that is being applied and compressing his windpipe with my right forearm. So all in all, he is not having a very good day! And I haven't finished yet!

This fast but interesting naked choke variation is shown in illustration 20, f. The curved white arrow indicates the direction that I have pushed the attacker's head with my left hand.

Illustration 20, f. The attacker is now being choked!

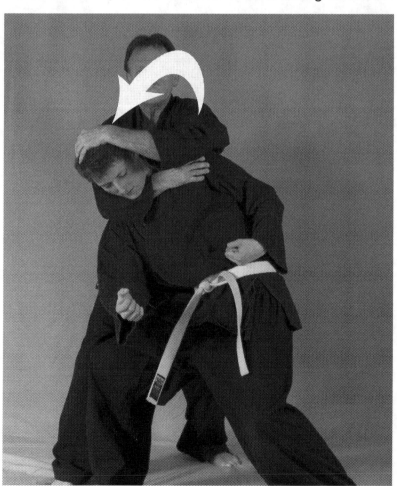

To conclude this **Hadaka jime** (naked neck lock) variation, using my left hand, I still keep the attacker's head tilted to his right shoulder, I then withdraw my arm from its throated arm bar, raise it upwards, then using my elbow, I strike downward into the attacker in the left trapezius muscle This is shown in illustration 20, f. The white straight arrow shows the direction of the elbow strike.

Illustration 20, f shows the conclusion to the **Hadaka jime** *(naked neck lock) variation routine.*

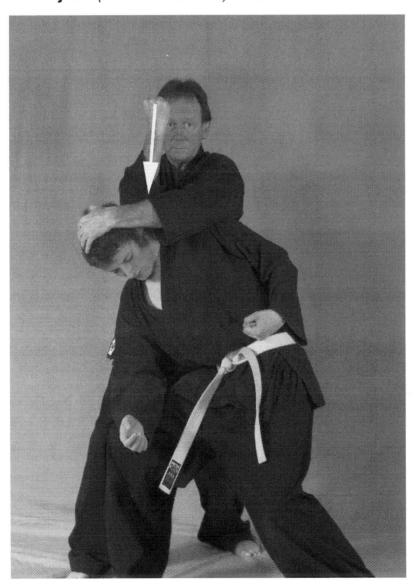

I know I'm nagging you, but if you try this routine, remember to practice both sides.

Okuri-Eri-Jime (送襟絞) Sliding collar neck lock.

In the next defence routine, I will utilise the attacker's jacket collar to apply a strangulation technique. This is a classic Shime-waza named, **Okuri-Eri-Jime** (送襟絞) Sliding collar neck lock.

For this routine, the attacker has a cosh in his right hand and his left leg forward. I have come into a fighting stance, left leg forward and as I have enough space, I have applied the "distance rule".

The distance rule is; If possible, keep the attacker at least one to two metres away from you; it makes it harder for him to attack you as he has further to lunge at you. This consequently makes the defence a little easer, as you have gained distance and be it a fleeting second, time.

Illustration 21, a shows the attacker armed and ready to attack.

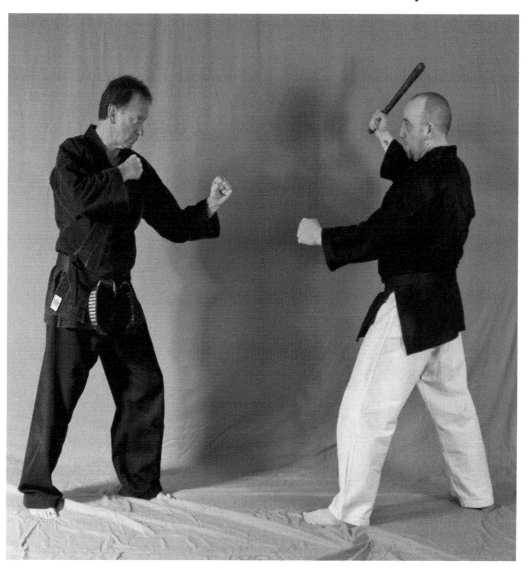

The attacker steps forward with his right leg and lunges at me with a side blow to the head. The large white curved arrow in illustration 21, b shows the direction of the attacker's intended strike. The white arrow on the floor indicates where he has stepped from.

To avoid having the side of my head caved in, I take a large step with my left leg and drop into a low forward stance. In conjunction with the step, I simultaneously duck under the attacker's right weapon arm and using my right palm heel, I strike the attacker upper torso to stun him. Note: To set up the sliding collar neck lock, the palm heel strike needs to be placed high so that the attacker does not collapse forward from the blow.

Illustration 21, b has a straight white arrow on the floor, this shows the direction of the step I have taken to duck under the attacker's right arm. The curved white arrow follows the direction my right hand has taken to deliver the palm heel strike.

Illustration 21, b. As the attacker lunges with a side blow, I duck and hit him with a palm heel strike.

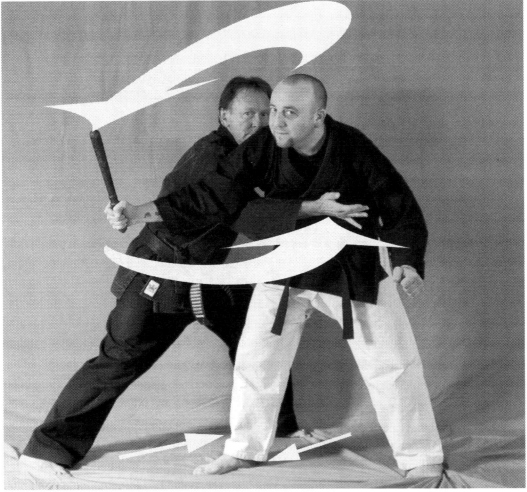

Note: Evading a side blow by ducking, takes time and practice to perfect as timing is critical for this manoeuvre. Start practicing slowly at first, then build up the attacking speed as you feel more confident.

With the attacker momentarily stunned from the palm heel strike, I need to do some more nifty coordinated movements.

I take a large step with my right foot, a small step with my left foot and then pivot on the ball of my feet. This puts me in a forward stance, facing the same direction as the attacker. These two steps are indicated in illustration 21, c, with two straight white arrows on the floor.

At the same time, using my left arm, I reach deeply around the front of the attacker's throat and using my left thumb, I slide it deep into the attackers collar, my four finger's then grasp the remaining cloth. This manoeuvre lines up the cutting edge of my forearm across the attacker's throat.

A split second after my left hand grasps the attacker's collar; I use my right hand, thumb to the inside, and grasp the attacker's left collar. Both of the actions are shown in illustration 21, c with two white curved arrows to help guide you through these movements.

In the left hand corner of the same illustration, I have included a small picture that shows how the thumbs are inserted in the inside of the attacker's collar, prior to taking a full hand grip.

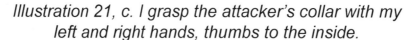

Illustration 21, c. I grasp the attacker's collar with my left and right hands, thumbs to the inside.

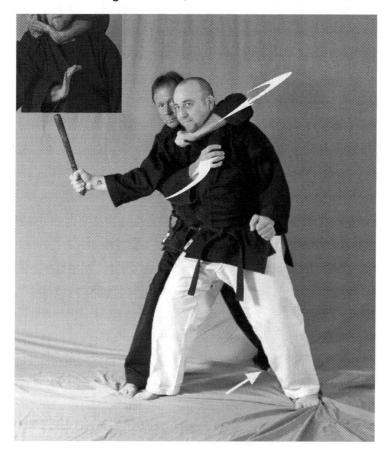

With my hands securely griping the attacker's collar, I then use my left hand to pull the attackers collar from my right to my left.

This manoeuvre has a dual purpose;

1) It draws the attacker off balance, so that his head rests on my left shoulder, this helps expose the throat area;

2) It also applies frontal pressure to the attacker's throat area by compressing the larynx and trachea.

Simultaneously, my right hand pulls the attacker's collar in the opposite direction, from my left to my right. To help guide you through intricate hand pulls, I have included two curved white arrows in illustration 21, d. I have also added two small photos that will help you understand the hand grips.

The **Okuri-Eri-Jime** (送襟絞) sliding collar neck lock acts like a hangman's noose, by combining these two pulling actions together, the neckline cloth tightens around the attacker neck! The result are; the larynx, trachea, carotid artery and jugular vein all being compressed at the same time!

Illustration 21, d shows the **Okuri-Eri-Jime**
(送襟絞) sliding collar neck lock being applied.

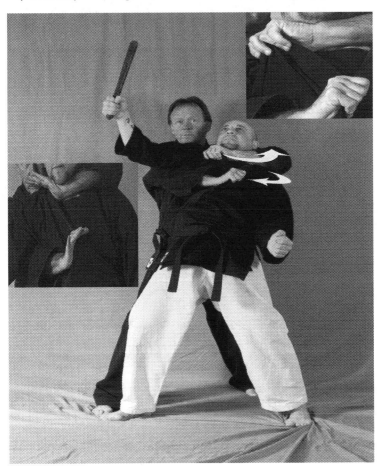

With the attacker subdued from the **Okuri-Eri-Jime** (送襟絞) sliding collar neck lock, I maintain control with my left arm and then release my right hand from its lower collar grip, fold the arm from its elbow joint, raise it high, then in one powerful action, I crash my elbow, atemi (当て身) into the attacker's right bicep; this will deaden the attacker's weapon arm while I prepare to finish this routine.

Illustration 21, e shows my right elbow smashing downward into the attacker's right bicep. The straight white arrow indicates the direction my elbow strike has travelled in.

Illustration 21, e. The attacker's weapon arm is struck in the bicep with a powerful elbow strike,

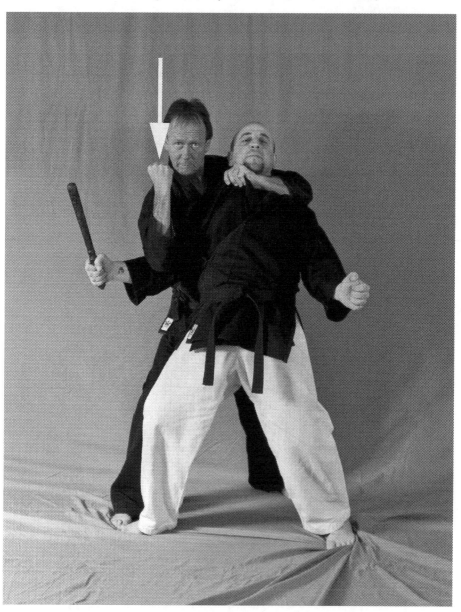

The final strike in this routine is what I call a rebound strike. A rebound strike happens a fraction of a second from the last strike. To understand this, let's back track to the last elbow strike.

As my right elbow crashes into the attacker's bicep, I pivot sharply to my left, dropping into a strong left side forward stance. In the same motion, I pull sharply to my left with my left hand; this draws the attacker off balance to his left side, exposing the attacker's right jaw line.

I then use the downward energy of the elbow strike as a rebound and immediately covert it into another strike. The strike I have used is a powerful jaw crunching lower knuckle reverse punch that lands on the attacker's right jaw line. The lower knuckles are used due to the angle of the jaw line.

This rebound lower knuckle reverse punch to the attacker's right jaw, is shown in illustration 21, f with three white arrows to help guide you through the final striking action.

*Illustration 21, f shows the conclusion to the **Okuri-Eri-Jime** (送襟絞)*
sliding collar neck lock routine with a reverse punch to the attacker's jaw,

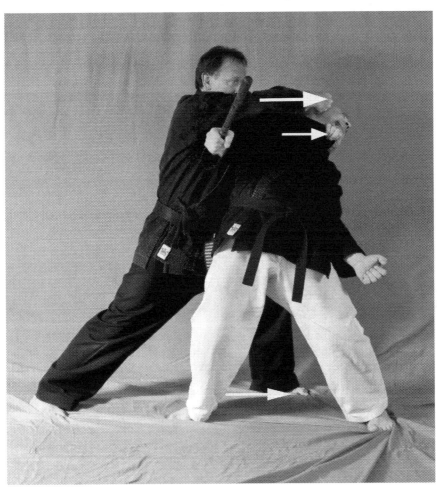

Don't forget to practice this technique both sides.

Kata-Ha-Jime (片羽絞). Single wing choke, or single wing neck lock.

The Kata-Ha-Jime (片羽絞) is an interesting strangulation technique (shime-waza) as it combines the usage the attacker's collar cloth and the "naked principle". That is, using ones hand for leverage to assist in applying the strangulation technique and not the cloth.

If you are confronted with a potential attacker out in the street, it is my first rule of engagement to come into a fighting stance, guard up; this is why at the start of each defence routine I show myself ready in a fighting stance, guard up. This is a rule you should adopt and never break.

The Kata-Ha-Jime (片羽絞) single wing choke will stick to this rule; both I and the potential attacker have come into a fighting stance, with our left legs forward. I have set the distance rule to a little over a meter, this means that when the attacker initiates his attack, he will have to lunge at me.

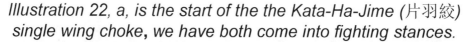

Illustration 22, a, is the start of the the Kata-Ha-Jime (片羽絞) single wing choke, we have both come into fighting stances.

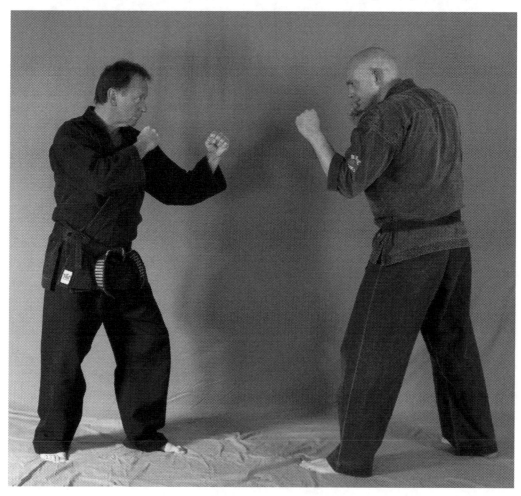

The attacker steps forward with his left leg to close the striking distance. In the same movement, he aims a reverse upper cut to my jaw with his right fist.

To avoid the upper cut, I quarter step to my left, ending up in a strong left forward stance. At the same time, using my right open hand, I parry this under the attacker's striking arm and then deflect the upper cut upwards.

These movements are shown in Illustration 22, b. The two white arrows on the floor indicate how I and the attacker have stepped forward. Looking at the attacker's right arm, the curved white arrow on it shows the direction of his intended upper cut punch, the same arrow indicates that his arm has been deflected upward. Looking below the attacker's arm is another curved white arrow; this indicates the route my right deflecting arm has taken.

Illustration 22, b. The attacker tries to punch me with an upper cut. I avoid it with a quarter step.

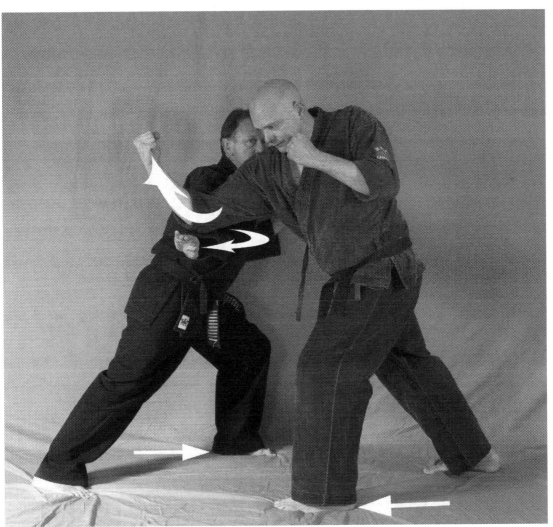

From my forward stance, I pivot sharply on the ball of my feet; this puts me facing the same direction as the attacker. To help you understand this foot pivot, I have included two small curved arrows on the floor in illustration 22, c.

As I pivot, I continue to deflect the attacker's right arm upward with my right arm. As my right hand passes past the attacker's right shoulder, I hook it around the back of the attacker's head and place my open palm on the back of the attacker's head. At the same time, I raise my left arm up, ready for the next part of the strangulation technique.

Illustration 22, c, shows my right open hand on the back of the attacker's head, the curved white arrow indicates the direction it has taken. The other large curved white arrow indicates the route that my left hand is taking in readiness for the next part of this technique.

Illustration 22, c. My right hand is placed on the back of the attacker's head.

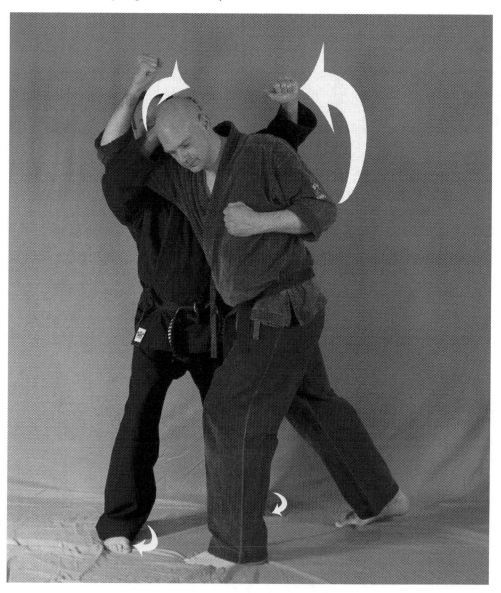

My left hand reaches around the front of the attacker's throat. Then using my left hand, thumb first, I grasp the right side of the attacker's collar.

Inserting the thumb first into the attacker's collar aligns the cutting edge of my forearm across the attacker's windpipe, a quick pull backwards instantly cuts off the attacker's airway.

Illustration 22, d shows my left hand taking a hold of the attacker's collar. The white curved arrow indicates the direction my left hand has travelled in.

Illustration 22, d. My left hand takes a grip of the right side of the attacker's collar.

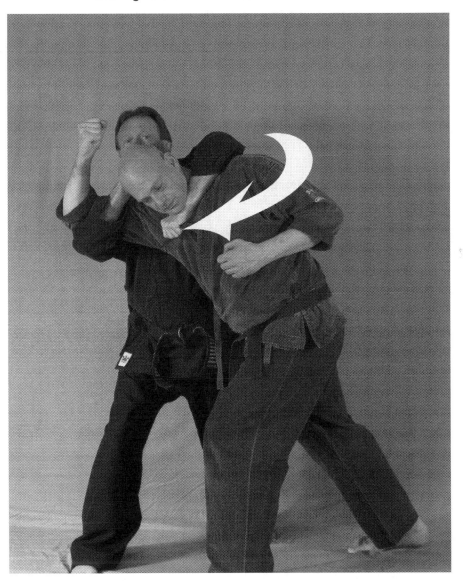

I now have every thing in place; the Kata-Ha-Jime (片羽絞) single wing choke is applied quickly by pushing forward with my right hand and at the same time, pulling backward and from right to left with my left hand. The result is the larynx, trachea and carotid artery are compressed and this strangles the attacker.

These two hand actions are shown in illustration 22, e with two white curved arrows to help you understand the mechanics of the hand movements. I have also added two small photo's in each corner of illustration 22, e that gives you different camera angles of the technique being applied.

*Illustration 22, e the **Kata-Ha-Jime** (片羽絞) single wing choke is being applied to the attacker.*

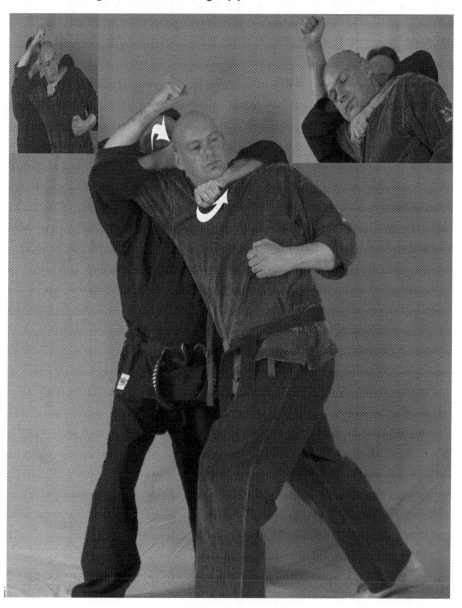

Keeping the single wing choke on, I push downward with my right hand, this breaks the attacker's balance by pushing him forward. Then in a simultaneous movement, with my right knee, I knee kick the attacker in his solar plexus.

These movements are shown in illustration 22, f with added arrows the help guide you through the movements.

Illustration 22, f. Using my right knee, I knee kick the attacker.

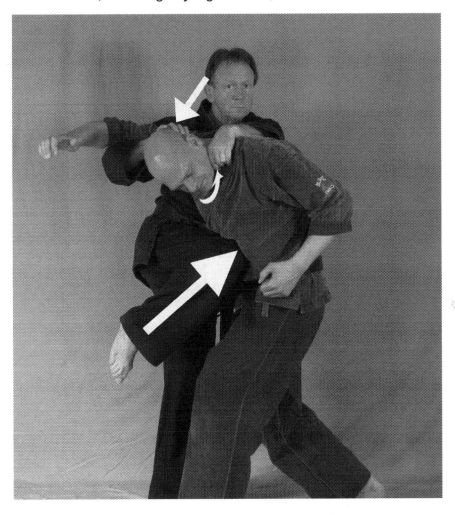

I am now ready to finalize this routine. As the knee kick impacts into the attacker's solar plexus, it causes the attacker to react by bending forward. I respond by replacing my right foot back on the floor and immediately adopt a right forward stance. In the same motion, I release my left hand from its collar grip, raise it upwards and then elbow strike the attacker on the nape of his neck.

The elbow strikeis shown in illustration 22, g with a white arrow added to indicate the direction on the elbow strike.

*Illustration 22, g shows the conclusion of the **Kata-Ha-Jime** (片羽絞) single wing choke with an elbow strike to the nape of the attacker's neck.*

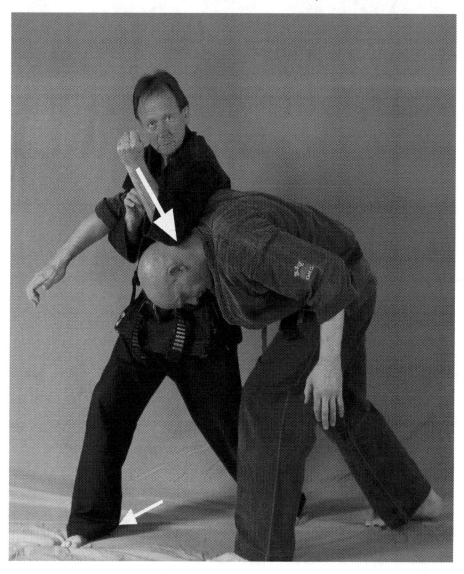

As always, once you are familiar with this technique on side, switch over and practice it on the other side.

Double sided neck vice strangulation.

I want to move away from some of the classic strangulations that are easily recognisable in both the Ju-Jutsu and Judo world and show you a true, blue blooded Ju-Jutsu strangulation technique. To my knowledge it has no reference name, so I will call it the double sided neck vice strangulation.

To illustrate the double sided neck vice strangulation, both I and the potential attacker have come into a left sided fighting stance with our guards up. I have applied the distance rule of keeping a least one metre away from the attacker. This is shown in illustration 23, a.

Illustration 23, a. The attacker and I have come into a fighting stance.

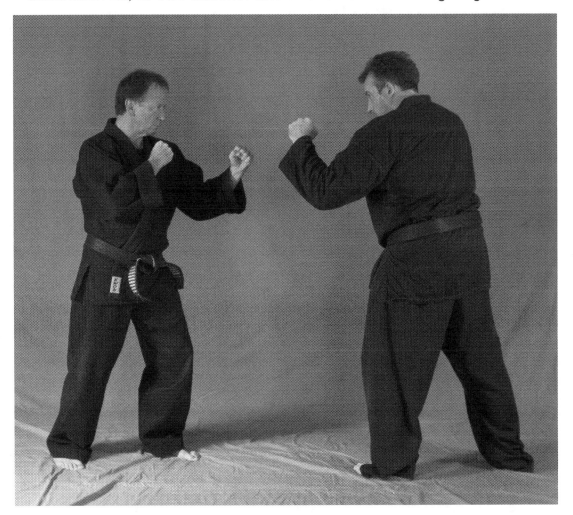

The attacker is a powerfully built man, he steps forward with his right leg and at the same times throws a big powerful right round house punch to the side of my head. His intention is to re-arrange my good looks!

With such a powerful blow, I need an equally powerful block to stop him dead in his tracks. The reverse outside forearm block fits this occasion well. From my fighting stance, I step directly to my left with my left foot. As I step, I forcibly swing my right arm from my right to my left allowing the edge of my forearm (ulna bone) to strike into the centre of the attacker's right forearm. If this technique is done properly, it could break the attackers forearm!

Illustration 23, b shows the attacker's right arm being blocked with a reverse outside forearm block. From the attacker's prospective, the white arrow on the floor indicates the step he has taken with his right foot and the curved white arrow shows the direction he is swinging his round house punch. From my prospective, the white arrow on the floor shows which way I have stepped with my left leg and the curved arrow indicates the swinging action I have employed to execute the reverse outside forearm block.

Illustration 23, b. The attacker's round house punch has been blocked with a reverse outside forearm block.

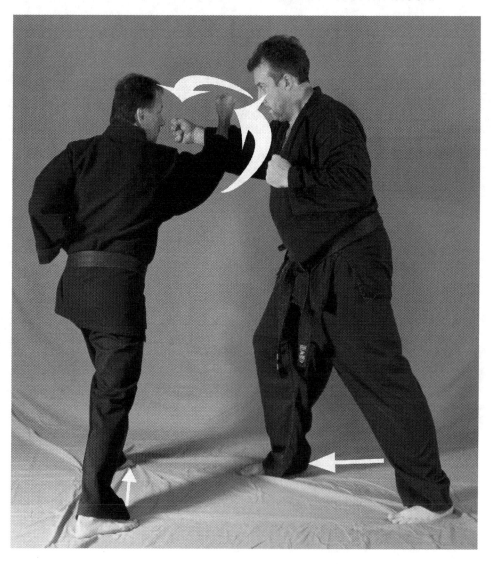

While the reverse outside forearm block has given the attacker something to think about (extreme pain) I pivot sharply on the ball of my feet and change from a left forward stance to a right forward stance. At the same time, I use a rebound technique and swing my right arm from left to right, striking the attacker on the right side of his neck. My own striking contact point is the edge of my outside forearm (ulna bone). This is an extremely powerful atemi (当て身) that can render the attacker immediately unconscious! So try to use this blow to stun the attacker rather than comatose him!

Illustration 23, c shows the outside forearm strike landing on the side of the attacker's neck, the curved white arrow indicates the direction of the strike. The two small curved arrows on the floor indicate the sharp pivot actions taken with my feet.

Illustration 23, c . The attacker is struck with an outside forearm strike to the right side of his neck.

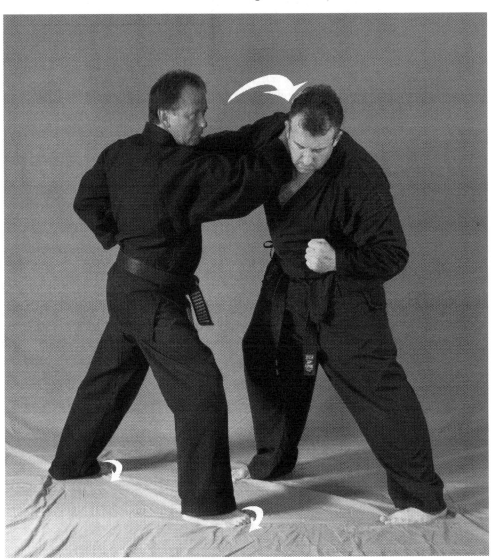

With the outside forearm strike stunning the attacker. I use my left arm to follow through with yet another powerful atemi strike. This is an unusual hook strike that crashes into the nape of the attacker's neck and drives his head forward. Yeah, you may have guessed it; this is another knock out blow! So moderate your striking power and use it to stun and subdue the attacker.

As the attacker's head drops from the hook strike, I use my right hand and grab hold of my left upper arm. My right hand now clamps onto the area around my left bicep and triceps muscles and the edge of my right forearm is cutting into the side of the attacker's neck. This compresses the attacker's right jugular vein and immediately affects the blood and oxygen supply to the brain.

These movements are shown in illustration 23, d. The large curved white arrow indicates the direction my left arm has travelled in to execute the hook strike. The small white arrow indicates my right hand is taking a hold of my left upper arm.

Illustration 23, d. The attacker is struck with a hook strike to the nape of his neck.

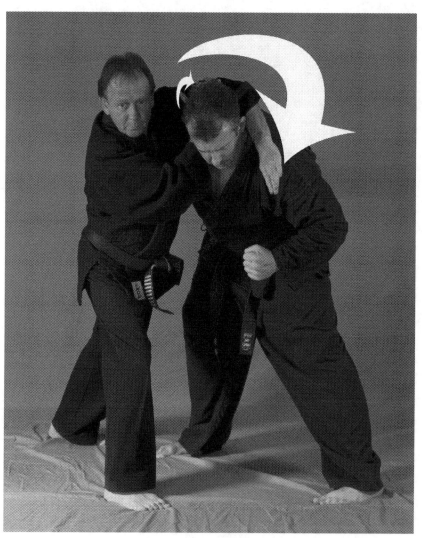

As the hook strike takes affect, I pivot sharply on left foot. At the same time, I push upwards with my right forearm and switch my body weight to my left side, this pushes the attacker upright.

As the attacker becomes upright, I keep my right hand in place on my own left upper arm and compress both sides of the attacker's neck by drawing both arms towards each other. This action is similar to a vice closing inward, the effect is the jugular vein is compressed. This causes cerebral ischemia and the attacker is well on the way to passing out! The double sided neck vice strangulation is now being applied. **Caution: Do not keep this strangulation on for more than a few seconds.**

The double sided neck vice strangulation is shown in illustration 23, e. The white curved arrow pointing to my right arm indicates the direction I used to push the attacker upright. The small curved white arrow on the floor indicates the shifting of my body weight.

Illustration 23, e. The double sided neck vice strangulation is being applied to the attacker.

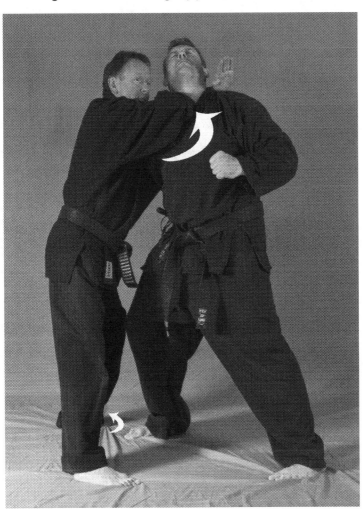

Ju-Jutsu techniques and self defence routines only work by setting the attacker up correctly, my next atemi strike is a prime example of this. The attacker has been pushed upright while the double sided neck vice strangulation has been applied; however this has left him defenceless for the next strike, a knee kick to the solar plexus. What a great setup!

I disengage my arms from the double sided neck vice strangulation and with as much power as I can muster; I crash my right knee into the attacker's solar plexus. This atemi is shown in illustration 23, f. The straight white arrow indicatives the direction my knee kick has travelled in.

Illustration 23, f. The attacker is knee kicked in the solar plexus.

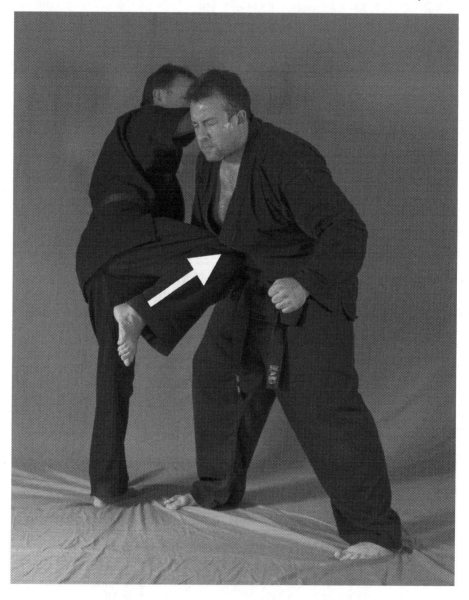

A kiai can be added at this stage for more power.

With the attacker heavily winded from the knee kick, I use the recoil from the impact of the knee kick and immediately step backward with my right leg. At the same time, I draw my right arm back and close my fist. My left hand supports the attacker's shoulder, this helps stop him collapsing forward.

Illustration 23, g shows the attacker being set up a reverse punch by me stepping backward with my right leg and aligning my right fist. I have included two white arrows that help explain these actions.

From the attacker's prospective, the realisation of what is going to happen next might be dawning on him! This is a classic set up!

Illustration 23, g. The attacker's life flashes in front of his eyes as I prepare to strike him!

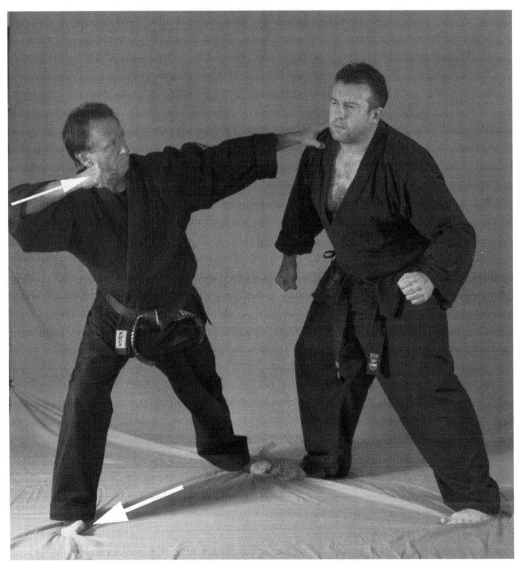

The conclusion of the double sided neck vice strangulation will not be a surprise to you........ or the attacker. Using my right fist, I strike the attacker with a powerful reverse punch (gyaku tsuki) on his chin. To add maximum power, I have co-ordinated the reverse punch with a fast stance change from my back leg to forward leg (前屈立ち *zenkutsu-dachi*). Illustration 23, h shows this final technique with a very spectacular photograph.

*Illustration 23, h draws a conclution to the the double sided neck vice strangulation routine with a jaw crunching (**gyaku tsuki**) reverse punch.*

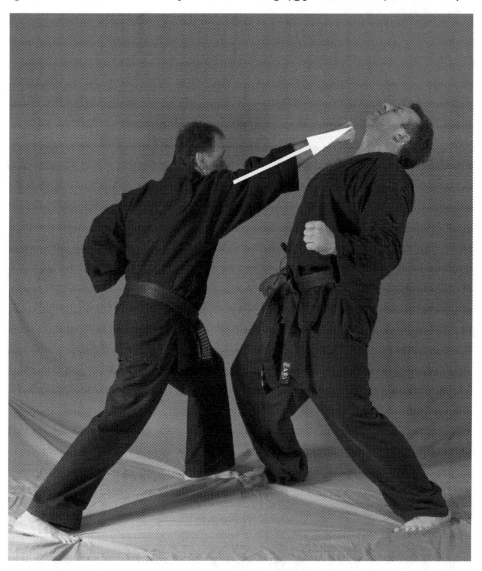

When you try this routine, practise it on both sides and add a kiai to the reverse punch (gyaku tsuki). Also remember, if this were a real attack out in the street, you need to come into a fighting stance once you have completed the defence routine............ just in case other attacker's want to join in the fun!

Reverse Hadaka jime (naked neck lock).

The final (**Shime-waza**) strangulation technique incorporated into a defence routine I want to show you is a **reverse Hadaka jime** (naked neck lock). From a Ju-Jutsu point of view, this is a classic strangulation technique that has a real place in all Ju-Jutsu and self defence syllabi. I have also seen this technique utilised in the U.F.C, cage fights and similar contests with great effect and in some cases it has resulted in an immediate submission.

To start this routine, illustration 24, a shows that both I and the attacker have come into a fighting stance, guards up with our lefts legs forward. I have adopted the distance rule and am just a little over a metre away from the attacker. When the attacker wants to attack me, he will now have to make up that distance; this will give me vital time to respond.

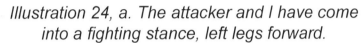

Illustration 24, a. The attacker and I have come into a fighting stance, left legs forward.

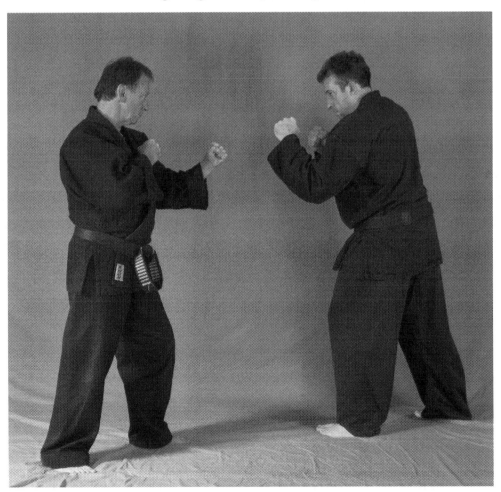

The attacker decides to go for it; he steps forward with his right leg and throws a big, powerful, right fisted round house blow to the left side of my face.

To block of his attack, I instantly extend my left sided fighting stance into a strong left sided forward stance, at the same time, in a powerful motion, I swing my left arm from right to left and block the attackers forearm with an outside forearm block. This block stops the attacker's arm dead! A powerful and well executed outside forearm block will at a minimum stun the attackers arm with pain, it could also break the attacker forearm!

These attack and defence movements are shown in illustration 24, b. To help you follow this, the smaller white curved arrow indicates the direction the attacker has thrown his round house punch in. The larger curved white arrow follows the direction of my left blocking arm. Looking down by my feet, the straight white arrow indicates my step from a fighting stance into a forward stance.

Illustration 24, b. The attackers tries to strike the side of my face with a round house punch but, his attack is stop dead by a powerful outside forearm block.

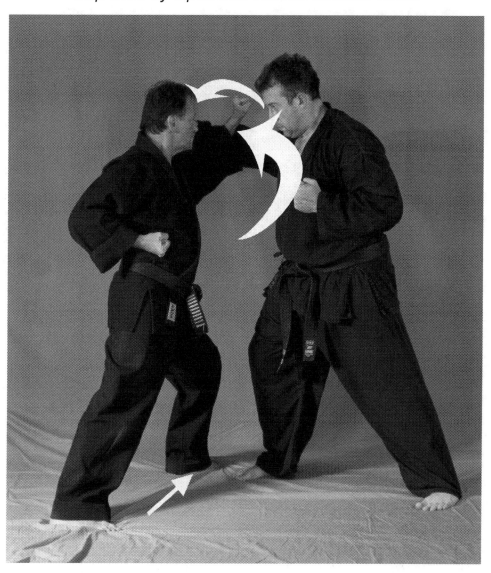

While the attacker is momentarily distracted from the outside forearm block, I give him something else to think about, a right elbow strike into his solar plexus.

The elbow strike is utilised for two reasons, firstly, it loosens up the attacker and secondly, the set up. As the elbow strike lands, it couses the attacker to fold forward as he is winded. The action of him folding forward will allow me to reach comfortably around his neck to strangle him.

Illustration 24, c shows the attacker being hit in the solar plexus with a right elbow strike (empi tsuki). This elbow strike (empi suki) is also an atemi.

Illustration 24, c shows the attacker being hit in the solar plexus with an elbow strike.

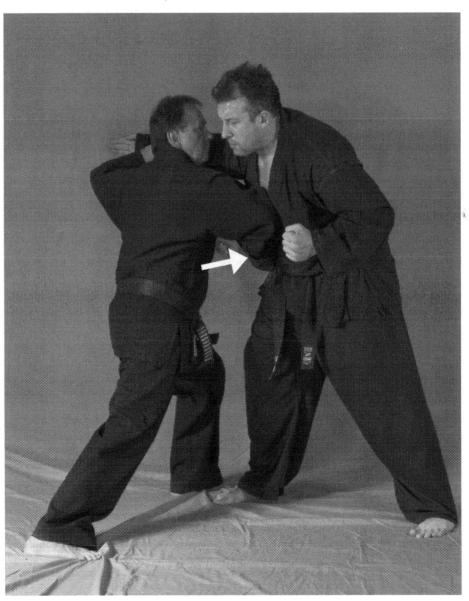

As the attacker folds forward from the elbow strike, I pop him with another elbow strike into the right side of his jaw. You may think this is an overkill but, in my books (excuse the witticism), it is better to be safe than sorry. Sorry is when you underestimate someone. That someone could be loaded with all kinds of drugs and alcohol! This will result in the nervous system and pain receptors shutting down and consequentially the attacker may not respond to some of the strikes and locks you apply…………Putting this elbow strike in makes you safe, not sorry.

Illustration 24, d shows the attacker being struck with a right elbow strike (empi tsuki) to the right side of his jaw. The straight white arrow indicates the elbows striking direction.

Illustration 24, d. The attacker is hit with a second elbow strike (empi tsuki), this time to the jaw.

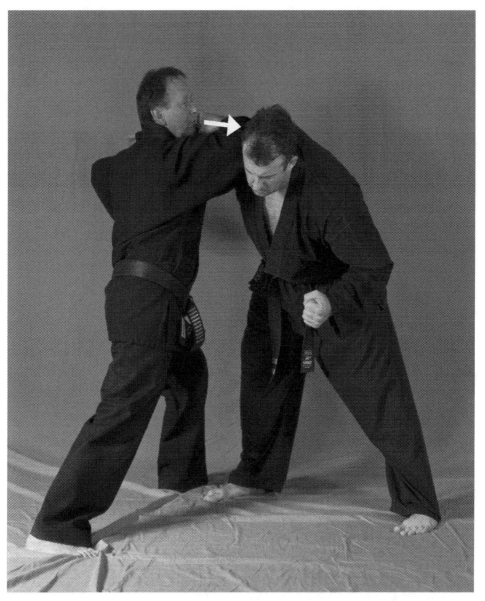

From the elbow strike to the attackers jaw, I unfold my right arm and then reach it over the back of the attackers head. This starts to draw the attacker forward and off balance, it also draws the attacker's head under my right arm pit. This is important as it is positioning his head for the impending reverse strangulation technique.

Illustration 24, e shows my right arm reaching around the back of the attacker head. The curved white arrow indicates the direction my right arm has travelled in.

Illustration 24, e. The attacker's head is drawn forward
by me reaching around the back of his head.

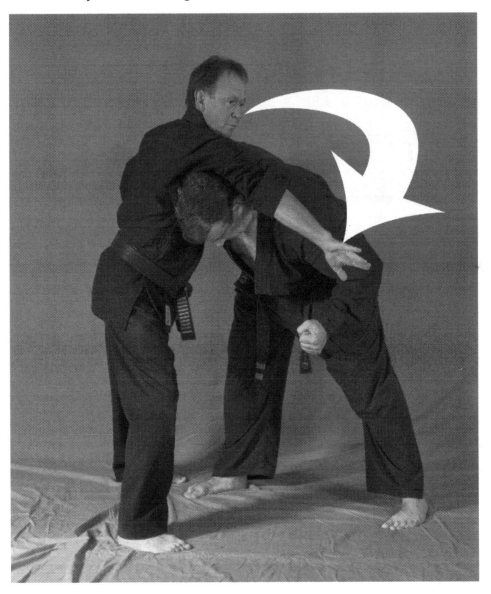

Continuing with my right arm swing I fold my arm and then hook it around the front of the attacker's throat, aligning the right edge of my right forearm (radius bone) with the attacker's windpipe.

I then grasp my right hand with my left. At the same time, I take a deep step back with my right leg and lever upwards. This applies the reverse **Hadaka jime** (naked neck lock). The effect is the attacker's larynx, trachea and carotid arteries are compressed. On the opposite side of the attacker's neck, extreme pressure is also being applied between the atlas and axis vertebras. The atlas is the topmost vertebra, and – along with the Axis – forms the joint connecting the skull and spine.

Illustration 24, f shows the reverse **Hadaka jime** (naked neck lock) being applied. The curved white arrow indicates the final direction my right arm has taken. Looking down to the floor, the straight white arrow indicates my step backwards. The two small pictures in the left and right corners have been added to help you understand the intricate hand and arm positioning. Study them well.

*Illustration 24, f. The reverse **Hadaka jime** (naked neck lock) is being applied the attacker.*

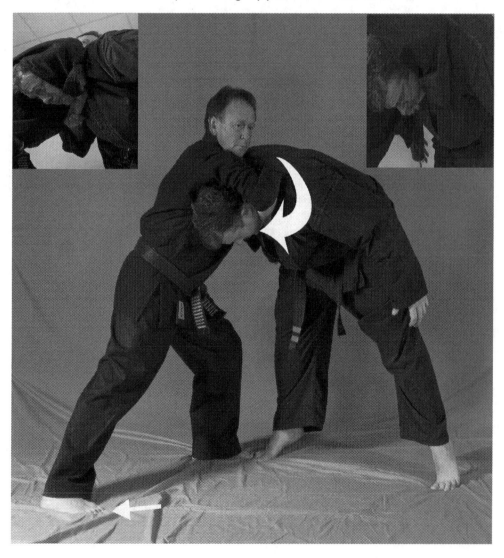

With the attacker "subdued" from the front reverse **Hadaka jime** (naked neck lock), *I have to admit, he does look a little worse for wear! See illustration 24, f.* I disengage my hands from around his neck and in a smooth action with my left hand, palm facing upwards I grasp a hold of the attacker's windpipe with my thumb and first finger. As well as crushing the windpipe, this stops the attacker from collapsing forward and supports his head for the final strike.

I then, in simultaneous movements, step back with my right leg and draw my right arm back ready to fire out the final blow. These movements are shown in illustration 24, f with arrows to help guide you through the various actions.

Illustration 24, f. The attacker is being set up for the final strike.

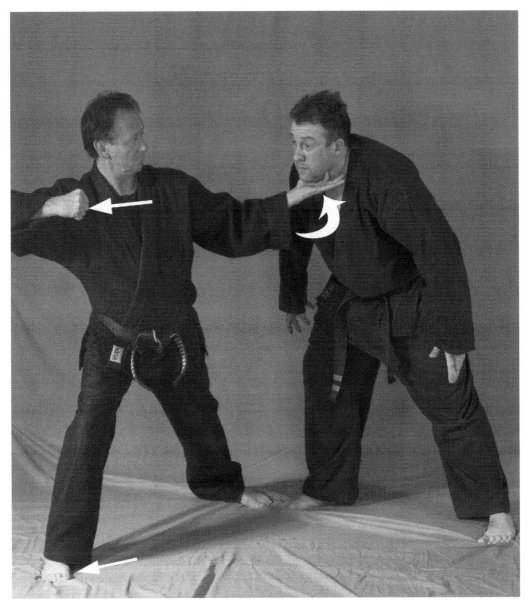

To conclude this reverse **Hadaka jime** (naked neck lock) defence routine In one smooth powerful action, I switch my body weight from my back leg to my forward leg; this puts me in a strong left sided forward stance (前屈立ち **zenkutsu-dachi**). And in a coordinated movement, using my right fist, I execute a powerful, teeth shattering reverse punch (gyaku tsuki) to the attacker on the chin.

The final punch (gyaku tsuki) of the routine is shown in illustration 24, g. The straight white arrow on my arm indicates the direction the punch has travelled in.

*Illustration 24, g. Shows the conclusion to the reverse **Hadaka jime** (naked neck lock) with the attacker being punched on the chin.*

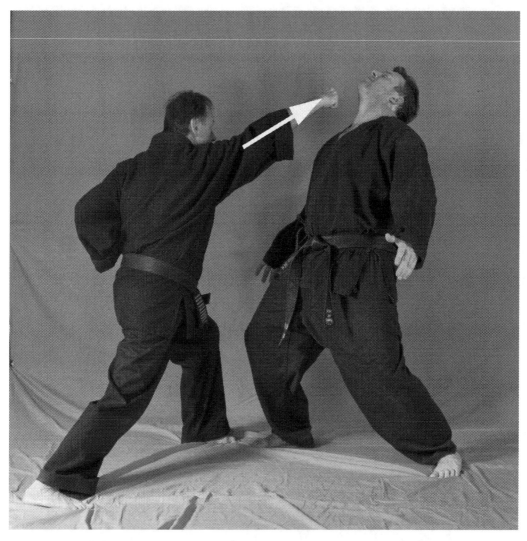

Caution: The reverse **Hadaka jime** (naked neck lock) is an extremely powerful strangulation technique. When you practice this, don't bang it on your training partner or lever upwards to sharply, it will only result in injury and a serious reprimand from your Sensei (teacher). Also remember to practice the **Hadaka jime** (naked neck lock) defence routine on the right and left sides.

Before I leave the strangulation techniques, I want you to be aware that the techniques demonstrated in this book have been done in a standing mode only. With a bit of ingenuity, you could easily adapt them for floor attacks defences and ground work grappling.

Self-defence and unarmed combat.

I have now covered what I class as the elementary basics of a Ju-Jutsu class. The area I now want to move to is a highly complex subject, the art of self defence and unarmed combat.

You may be a little bewildered and think, well what were all the previous techniques in this book about? Attacks were coming in and defences were applied in great length. Aren't they self defence? Well, yes they are, but I was concentrating on specific areas of Ju-Jutsu, atemi, locks, throwing methods and strangulation techniques. I now need to add other techniques so that you the reader can get a true overall picture of Ju-Jutsu and the unique way it deals with self defence.

The definition of self defence is the act of defending oneself, one's property or the well-being of another from physical harm. This statement may sound cut and dry but when one really looks at all the different ways a person or persons can be attacked, you begin to understand the enormity and complexity of the art of self defence and unarmed combat. This complex issue has been addressed by many of the founding fathers of Ju-Jutsu and unarmed combat arts. What each has believed on the subject is that there are no easy answers. A student of this must be prepared to look at each attack, analyse it and then look at all the possible ways of implementing a successful defence and then master that or those techniques.

The body mechanics of an attack.

To analyse an attack, one must break the attack down into all its intricate components. This I call the body mechanics of an attack. To understand this, as an example only, let's take a punch to the face as the primary attack. The first thing to address is the overall size of the attacker; the taller they are the longer there striking reach will be. This can affect your initial defence. Next, what kind of punch is it? Is it a right or a left handed punch, this will affect the direction you move into or any block, parry or technique you use in your defence. Is the punch a jab, which will make it quick and snappy. Is it a lunge punch, slightly slower but more powerful. Is it a reverse punch, which is fast and powerful.

The analyses now has to go deeper, each strike listed above has its own body mechanics that makes that move possible, as each strike is different, It affects the defence strategy immensely.

Punching analyses in detail.

The jab punch. The characteristics of the jab are as follows; the attacker stands in a classic boxing or freestyle fighting stance, then the lead fist is thrown straight ahead and the arm is fully extended. Once the jab is thrown, the lead arm is retracted quickly. If he or she leads with the right then they will jab with the right, if they lead with the left, they will jab with the left. This is a short fast attack with a short based stance.

The lunge punch. The characteristics of the lunch punch are as follows; the attacker stands in a classic boxing or freestyle fighting stance and then lunges a punch at you with the leading arm, extending the arm fully. He or she also extends the same side leg into a long based forward stance. If he or she leads with the right then they will lunge with the right, if they lead with the left, they will lunge with the left. This is a medium speed attack, with a long strong based stance.

The reverse punch. The characteristics of the reverse punch are as folows; the attacker stands in a classic boxing or freestyle fighting stance and then steps forward with lets say the left leg into a deep forward stance and simultaneously throws a reverse punches with the right fist, extending the arm fully. If the attacker were doing this punch with the left hand, they would step forward with the right. This is a fast, powerful strike with a long strong based stance.

What can be deduced from the analyses is; the punches aimed to the face all have different power ratios and the stances differ according to the punch being thrown. What can also be deduced is the attacker will be off balance at different angles according to what stance he or she is in.

Before you can start to work on the defence of these attacks, you need to throw in a few more factors into the defence equation. The street environment - The attack terrain- Street Awareness.

The street environment.

The dojo (martial arts place of practice) is or should be a safe environment for practicing ones chosen martial art. The training area should be free from dangerous obstacles and equipped with the appropriate safety equipment.

The street environment where a real attack happens is full of obstacles, obstructions, hazards and other people who might want to join in the attack. Strategies have to be built into ones defence techniques to accommodate these street environmental normalities.

The attack terrain.

The attack terrain is the ground the attacker or attacker's stands on and initiates the attack. It could be a nice even carpeted surface or it could be a piece of waste land with building rubble everywhere and water filed pot holes. It could on grassy wet bank, a steep hill or in an unlit stair well. Once again strategies have to be built into the defence techniques to accommodate ones own footing and the tactics used in different terrains.

154

To address all of these issues, I teach each student a "minimum of three defences for each attack". One defence technique will deal with the attacker directly front on. The second will deal with the attacker's right side and the third with the attacker's left side. This way, you have a minimum of three defence options per attack. Now if you consider how many different ways you can be attacked, you are going to learn thousands of defence techniques.

Ok…I can see that you are thinking, this is tooooooooo complicated, how am I supposed to learn all of this?

It takes time and lots of practice. The English Channel tunnel wasn't built in a day. Your Ju-Jutsu, unarmed combat and self defence skills will take time to develop, you have to take one attack at a time, master the defence of that attack and then move on to the next one. Then periodically go back to the basics defences and practice them again, this time refining the defence techniques. This cycle is what makes an average martial artist a great martial artist, practice and then practice some more.

Street Awareness.

To start this section on self defence, we must first take our minds out of the dojo and think of attacks out in the street. The first lesson that we have to learn is street awareness. Street awareness is being alert to potential attacks and sticking to the "don't do list"

The "don't do list" is endless and it depends on your own personal lifestyle. To give you an example; don't flash your money, ipod, mobile phone and other expensive items around in public area's. Don't use cash machines if dodgy looking people are hanging around. Don't park you car in unlit areas. Don't leave your car door open when you are in it, (car-jacker's love this.) Don't walk down dark alleys on your own. I would seriously recommend that you look at your own life style and then make up your own "don't do list" as part of your own street awareness program.

Front strangulation attack and defence routine.

Even with the best "don't do list" in the world, we can still be taken by surprise. In the first attack, the attacker has been able to get past my initial distance rule by approaching me in a friendly manner and asking for the time, (it could have been for directions or numerous other clever ploys). He then surprises me with a sudden lunge into a front strangle attack! He has his left leg forward.

My immediate line of defence is to regain my lost posture from the impact of the attack. To do this, I step back with my right leg; this leaves me in a short left sided stance. I also tense my neck muscles to help resist the strangulation. This is shown in illustration 25, a.

I, and you also have to overcome the shock of being attacked. My key tip on this is; 'Train hard, fight easy'. You constantly have to incorporate a high degree of realism into your club training. This will help immensely in overcoming the initial attack shock factor and the attacker out in the street.

Illustration 25, a. The attacker grasps my throat and is trying to strangle me

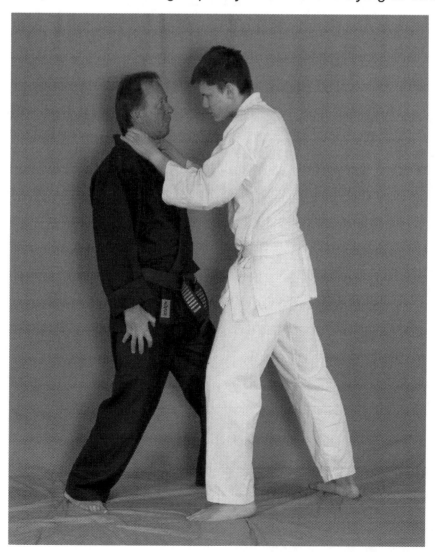

With any attack situation, I always employ a "positive mental attitude", P.M.A. The initial positive element of this particular attack is the attacker has tied up two of his major weapons, his hands. With his hands tied up, he is not able to throw any punches - P.M.A.

Once I have regained my posture, I take a big step past the attacker with my left leg; this is to the attacker's right side. I also coordinate the step with two simultaneous actions, my left palm heel is driven under attacker's chin knocking him backwards, and at the same time I use my right hand and grasp a hold of the attacker's waist belt and pull sharply towards me. From a street point of view, you can grab a hold of anything in "that area" that comes to hand! Use your imagination!!!

These actions are shown in illustration 25, b. If you look down toward the floor, the small white arrow indicates the step I have taken with my left leg. The straight white arrow on my arm indicates the direction of the palm heel strike. Looking at the attacker waist line, the curved black arrow indicates the pull towards me.

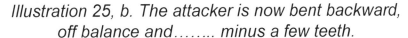

Illustration 25, b. The attacker is now bent backward,
off balance and…….. minus a few teeth.

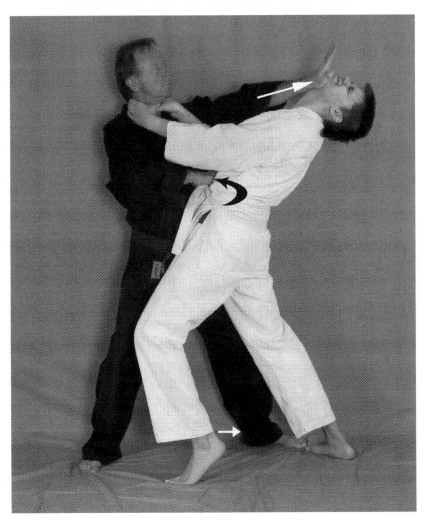

As my left palm heel strike under the attacker's chin runs out of striking power. I instantly convert it into a push and continue to drive the attacker further off balance.

At the same time, my right hand is still gripping the attacker's belt (or other parts out in the street!) and I use it to pull in the opposite direction to the palm heel push. The attacker is now so far off balance backwards, he resembles a champion limbo dancer!

Illustration 25, c shows the attacker been driven further off balance. The large curved white arrow indicates the direction of the push with my left hand; the small curved arrow indicates the pulling direction with my right hand.

Illustration 25, c. The attacker is driven off balance
with a strong left handed push under his chin.

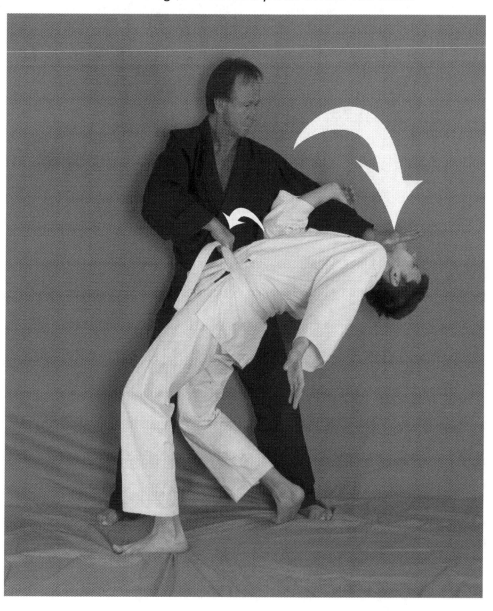

The attacker's body has now reached the point of no return. At this stage; I have released my right hand grip of the attacker's belt and allow the attacker to fall to the floor.

This is a simplistic Ju-Jutsu throw that works on a pull and push method. However if executed correctly the final body impact is devastating.

Illustration 25, d shows the attacker been thrown to the floor. Please note: Because the attacker is falling at such a great speed. It took several attempts and numerous lens recalibrations to capture this picture. My uke, (training partner) that was being constantly smashed to the floor was extremely relieved when we finally had an acceptable shot! Oh ok, I blinked but I hadn't the heart to put him through any more grief.

Illustration 25, d. The attacker is being thrown to the floor.

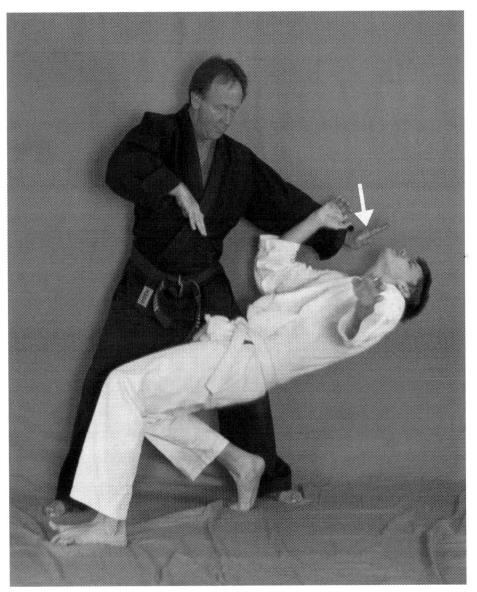

To finalise this front strangulation attack and defence routine, as the attacker hit the floor, using my right foot, I heel stamp kick him in the groin. A kiai can be added for more kicking power.

This heel stamp is shown in illustration 25, e. The straight white arrow indicates the direction of the heel stamp kick.

Illustration 25, e. The front strangulation attack and defence routine is concluded with a heel stamp kick to the groin.

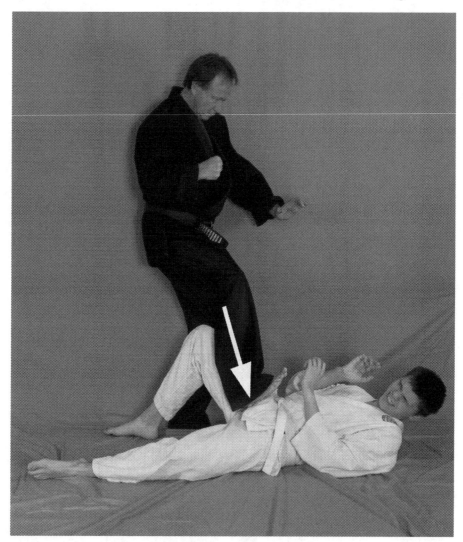

Taking into account what I have wrote about "the street environment" and "the attack terrain" you will now understand the added importance of practicing this defence routine both sides.

Finally, if this attack were out in the street, as soon as I heel kicked the attacker in the groin, I would immediately come into a fighting stance, ready to deal with any other potential attacker's.

Bear hug at the front, arms pinned attack and defence routine.

As much as don't like letting the attacker get too close, in the next attack, the attacker and I have ended up toe to toe! This is the reality of street attacks; I or any attack victims have little or no choice in the initial battle ground. The attacker will always have the upper hand on this and in most cases the element of surprise. What will surprise him is what comes next!

Illustration 26, a, shows the opening movement to the defence from a front bear hug, armed pinned with the attacker and I standing toe to toe in left fighting stances.

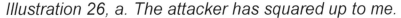

Illustration 26, a. The attacker has squared up to me.

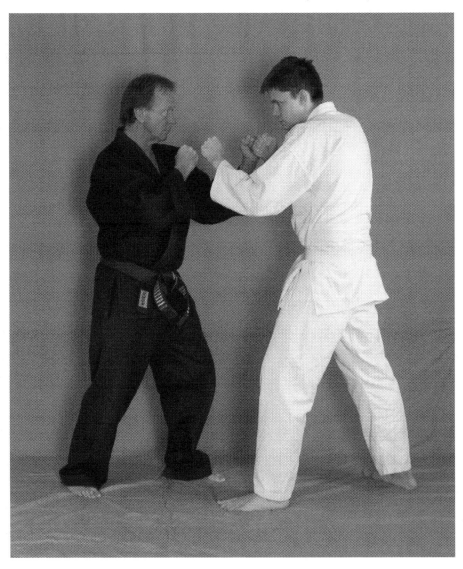

From his fighting stance, the attacker lunges at me and tries to pin both my arms with a strong bear hug hold.

To counter this attack, I step back with my right leg and drop into a deep, strong stance. At the same time, I shoot both arms out and brace my hands on the attacker's hips. As an extra precaution, I have shifted my head to my left side, this saves any accidental head collisions. These initial counter movements are shown in illustration 26, b with white arrows added to help you understand the attack and initial line of defence.

The combination of counter movements frustrates the attacker by making him reach and stretch to the point where his attack is weak. If I were to stand still and let him apply this hold, I would be in serious trouble; he or a stronger person could actually start to cave my ribs in! That's why the name "bear hug" for this attack is appropriate.

Illustration 26, b. The attacker tries to grab me in a "bear hug hold"

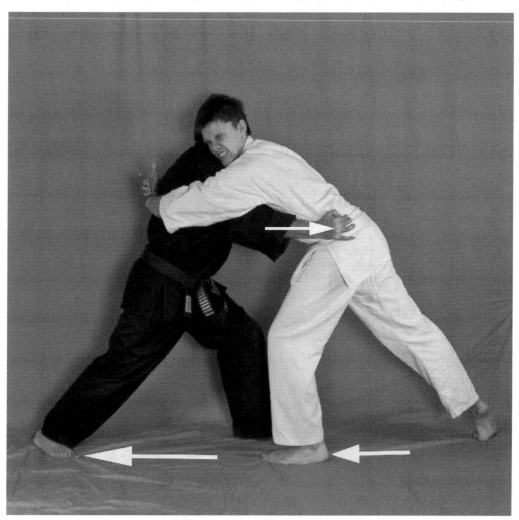

Keeping my hands on the attacker's hips to support his upper torso, I use my right knee and deliver a powerful knee kick into the attacker's solar plexus. This is shown in illustration 26, c. The large white arrow on my right leg indicates the route of the knee kick.

If you were doing this routine and the attacker is much taller than you, then a knee groin kick or lower stomach might be more appropriate.....and if the first one doesn't work, keep firing them out!

Illustration 26, c. The attacker is regretting attacking me!
His breakfast and dinner is now in his mouth, as I fire a
powerful right knee kick into his solar plexus.

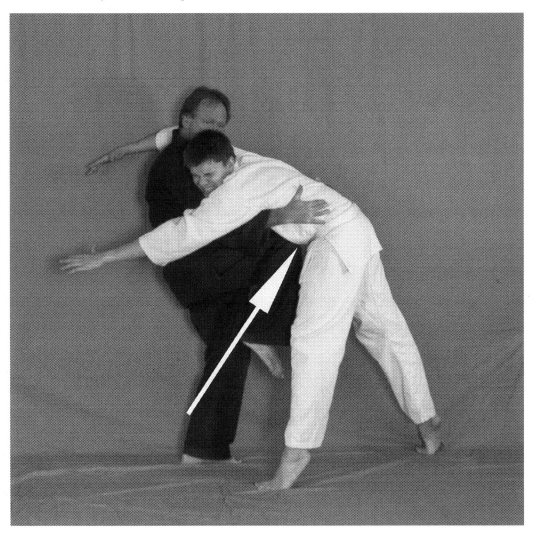

As soon as the right knee kick lands, I step back with my right leg and pivot to my right side. In a continuous flowing action, with the attacker's right arm resting on my left shoulder, I scoop my left arm around the back of the attacker's right shoulder and grasp the edge of my right hand with my left hand. This unbalances the attacker by drawing him forward, at the same time it applies a "mild" shoulder lock.

Illustration 26, d shows the attacker being drawn forward and a mild shoulder lock being applied. To help you understand the actions in this illustration, the straight white arrow pointing to my foot indicates my right foot has stepped back after the knee kick. The large curved white arrow indicates the route my right arm has travelled in and the small curved white indicates the action take with my left hand to grasp my right.

Illustration 26, d. The attacker's right arm is trapped on my left shoulder and he is being drawn off balance.

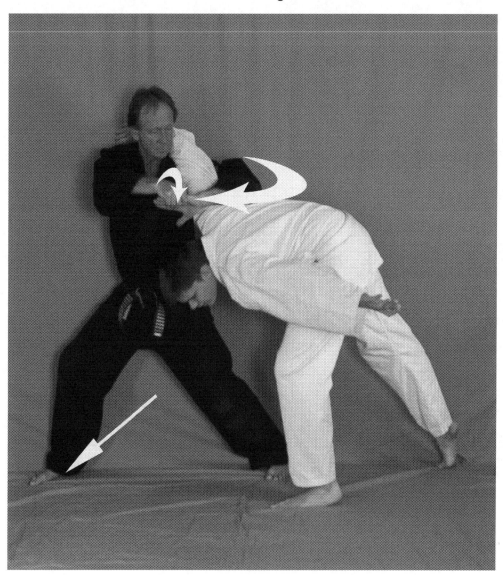

I continue to draw the attack off balance and drive him towards the floor. As he drops onto his left knee, I keep control of the attacker's shoulder with my left arm and let his right arm slide down the front of my chest, this allows his right arm to straighten. With the attacker's right arm now elevated upwards, the shoulder lock goes from mild to severe! These movements are shown in illustration 26, e.

Ilustration 26, e. The attacker collapses onto his left knee and his right shoulder is being locked.

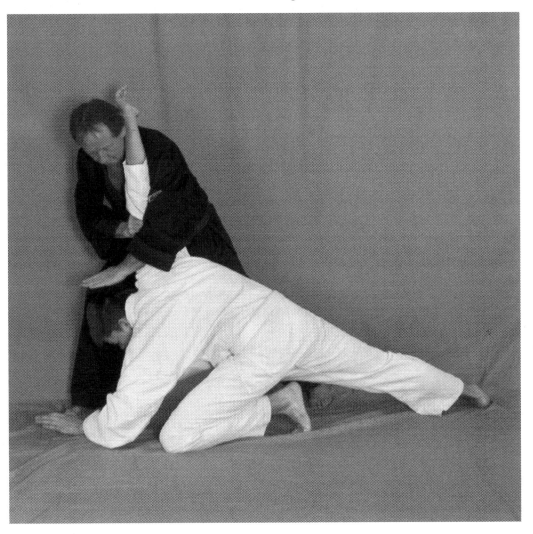

I keep the attacker's arm elevated upwards and drive him face down on the floor. Once he hits the floor, I crash my right knee in between his shoulder blades, this is an excellent striking point, and it also helps restrain him.

With the attacker immobilised, my left hand takes a hold of the attacker's right upper forearm and my right hand takes a hold of the attacker's hand. With the attacker's right arm, wrist and hand secured, I then turn everything clockwise. The result is an exceptionally painful wrist and shoulder lock, just look at the attackers face in illustration 26, f.......he's not acting! The small curved white arrow in this illustration will help you to understand the wrist and arm rotation. The arrow pointing down to my knee indicates the direction my knee has taken in order to pin the attacker painfully to the floor.

Illustration 26, f. The attacker is immobilised face down on the floor and restrained with a wrist and shoulder lock.

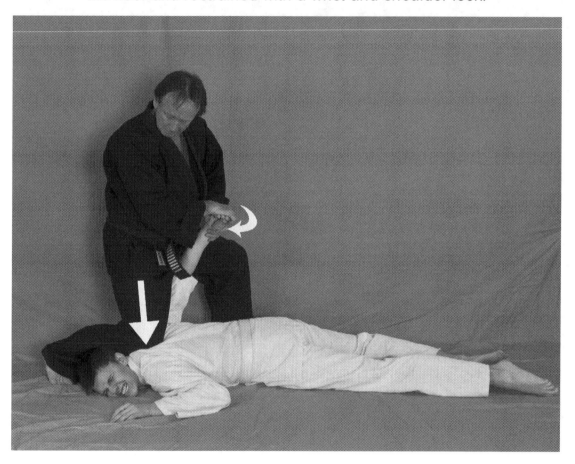

With the attacker nice and secure on the floor, I can plan my safe exit. Exit strategy is an essential part of any self defence routine.

The first part of my exit strategy is to make sure that the attacker is not capable of any immediate fight back when I release him from his restrained position. To do this, using my right fist, I strike him in his right kidney; this is another atemi point. This is shown in illustration 26, g. The straight white arrow indicates the direction my right arm has taken for the kidney punch.

Illustration 26, g. Before I release the attacker and to stop "fight back", I strike him in the kidney.

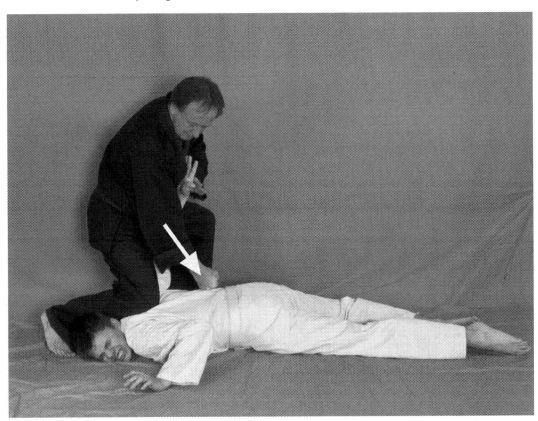

To conclude this defence routine, with the attacker stunned from my kidney shot, I release the wrist and shoulder lock and the stand up in a fighting stance. This is shown in illustration 26, h.

The fighting stance positioning I have taken has some tactical significance. The stance puts me just above the attacker's head; this allows me to keep an eye on him as I exit the area. It also gives me, fighting breathing space; fighting breathing space is the distance between me, the original attacker and any new attackers. An example of how this works is, I use the original attacker as an obstacle that makes it difficult for the next attacker or attacker's to get at me. By standing above the attacker's head and knowing that the potential attacker's will be approaching from the floored attacker's feet, it has given me have a minimum of six feet (1.75m) of fighting breathing space.

The next thing I need to do is plan my safe exit from this attack area. As a simple rule, I will exit where the least line of hostile resistance is. If this means having to change my route to avoid battling my way through half a dozen of the attacker's mates, then I take it. If the long way around is the safe way around, then that's my safe exit.

llustration 26, h. Shows the conclusion of the bear hug at the front, arms pinned attack and defence routine with the attacker being down and out!

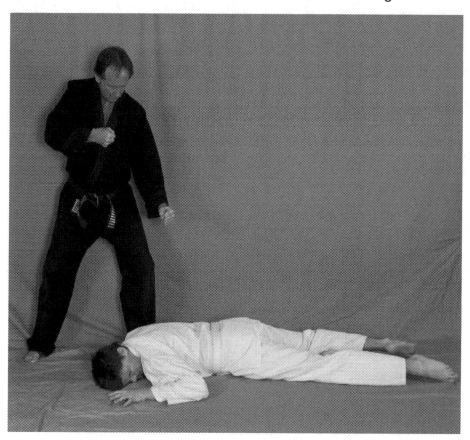

This is my third martial arts book; those who have read my previous books will by now understand my style of writing, my obsession with every small detail and that I repeat myself. This is my martial way, the way I train and teach. So once again I will happily repeat, once you have practiced this defence routine on one side and feel confident, change over and practice it the other side.

Rear strangulation and defence routine.

It would be nice to think all attacks came in from the front only; sadly the attacker is a cunning, devious creature. He or she knows only too well that attacking from the rear has the elements of both stealth and surprise. In the next attack, a strangulation from the rear, the attacker has moved stealthily up behind me and grabs me around the neck with both hand. His intention is to kill me!

My immediate reaction is a combination of movements, all done simultaneously: I do not panic, I tense my neck muscles to help resist the attack and I step back into the attacker with my right leg; this simple move throws the attacker off balance. These reactions and movements are shown in illustration 27, a. The straight white arrow on the floor indicates the direction I have stepped back with my right leg.

Illustration 27 a. The attacker is trying to strangle me
from the rear. I step back to break his balance.

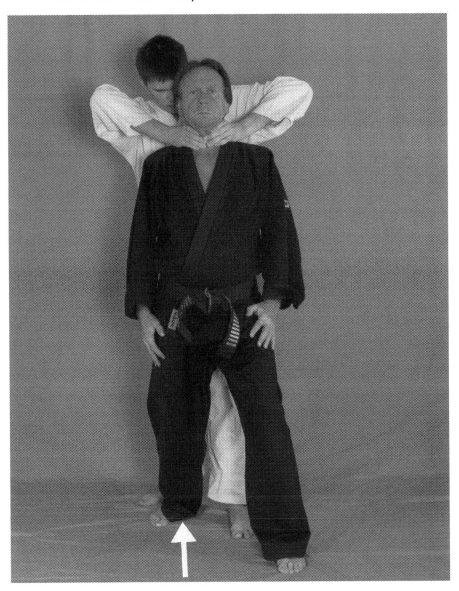

Now for a bit more of P.M.A. (positive mental attitude). In an attempt to strangle me, the attacker has put his hand around my neck, tying up two of his major weapons, his hands. The only area that he is restraining is my neck; this leaves the rest of my body free. With this in mind, I can move easily.

I reverse my right foot backwards but not in a straight line, look at the arrow on the floor in illustration 27, b, it looks like a letter 'L' with an arrow head and this is the route my right foot has taken. As the 'L' step is completed, I drop into a deep straddle stance. The 'L' route is taken to avoid my right foot colliding with the attacker's left foot.

As I am stepping backward, I close my right fist and place my left palm heel on the fist. Then, just as I drop into the straddle stance, I fire a powerful re-enforced elbow strike into the attacker's solar plexus; this is another atemi point. This striking movement is shown in illustration 27, b with a large curved white arrow indicating the route the re-enforced elbow strike travelled in.

Illustration 27, b. I step back into a straddle stance and re-enforce elbow strike the attacker in the solar plexus.

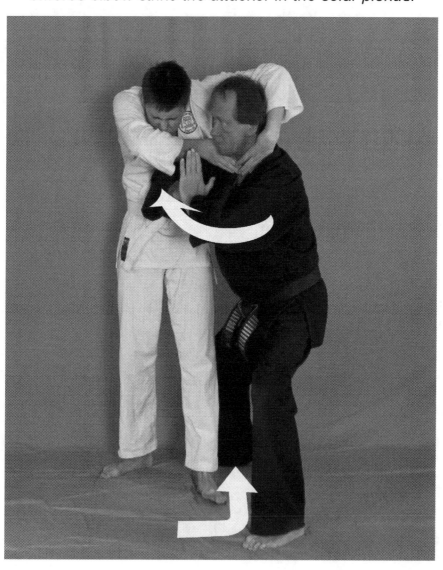

As the re-enforced elbow strike crashes into the attacker's solar plexus, the attacker responds by collapsing forward from his waist line. This is exactly what I want to happen. I then take advantage of this by effortlessly passing my right arm under the attacker's left arm pit and then hook it around his left shoulder. His left arm now rests on my right shoulder.

These actions are shown in illustration 27, c. The small black curved arrow in this illustration indicates the initial direction my right hand travelled in order to pass under the attacker's arm pit. The larger curved white arrow pointing to my hand indicates the route my right arm has taken as I reached around the attacker's left shoulder.

Illustration 27, c. I have hooked my right arm around the attacker's left shoulder.

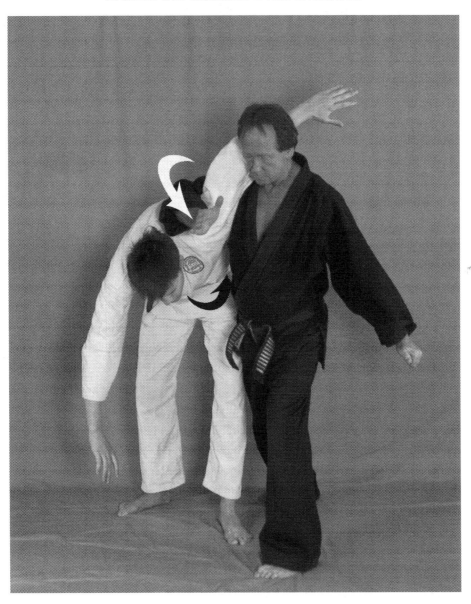

With the attacker's left arm secured, I pivot on the ball of my feet so that I am facing the attacker's left side, I then drop immediately into a left sided forward stance. This movement has allowed me to draw the attacker's left arm closer to my body, by scooping his shoulder toward me with my right arm; I can now apply a moderate shoulder lock.

It is quite natural for the attacker to try to fight back or to try to regain his posture by attempting to stand upright. To stop this, I strike the nape of his neck with a left forearm strike; this strike into his neck is another atemi point.

All of the above movements are shown in Illustration 27, d. The two small curved white arrows on the floor indicate the pivoting action I have taken to face the attacker's left side. The straight white arrow indicates the direction my forearm has travelled in order to strike the nape of the attacker's neck.

Illustration 27, d. The attacker's left shoulder is locked and he gets a good bash on the back of his neck from my left forearm.

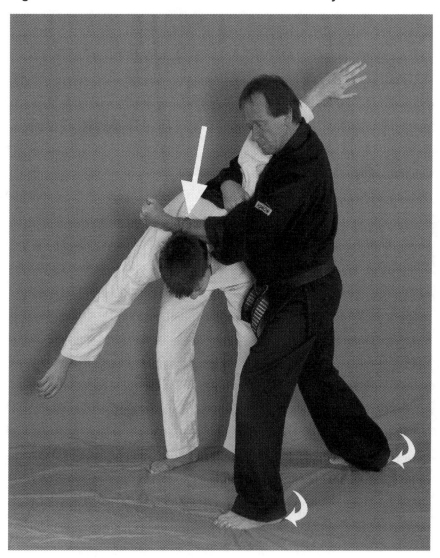

With the attacker stunned from the forearm strike, using my left hand, I reach around and grab a hold of the attacker's chin; I then rotate his chin clockwise. This applies a powerful neck and shoulder lock. This movement is shown in illustration 27, e. The curved black arrow indicates the direction that the attacker's chin is being turned.

Warning: care must be taken when trying this technique; you could quite easily break your training partner's neck!

Author's note: While others consider Ju-Jutsu as a sport, **"I Do Not".** The only game being played out here is the one of life or death. If you take a step back to the start of this attack, the attacker was trying to kill me; all I am doing is exercising my rights to defend myself. Any and all of the techniques I have explained so far in this book could injure the attacker severely. My answer to any attacker is, I know Ju Jutsu, leave me alone and I will leave you in peace, attack me and I will leave you in pieces.

Illustration 27, e. One of Ju-Jutsu's most powerful neck locks is being applied to the attacker.

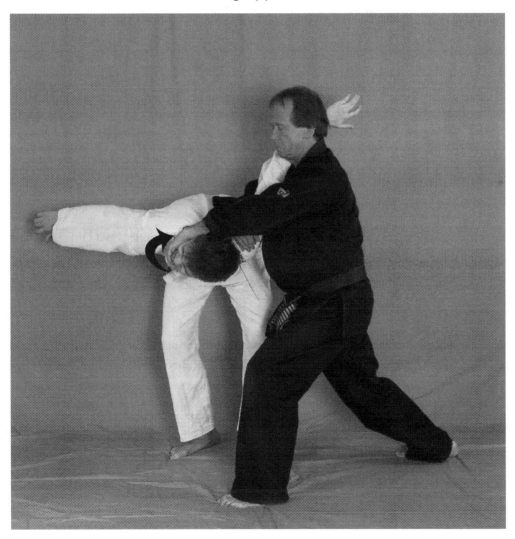

While keeping the neck and shoulder lock on the attacker, I raise my right knee upward and knee kick the attacker in the left side of his jaw, this strike is another atemi point. From a self defence point of view, I always class a knee kick as one of the last kicks I teach my students, not the first. The reason is you have to be in close to deliver this kick, sometimes other longer ranged kicking techniques are safer to deliver. In this case, it is safe to do this kick as the attacker is in a restrained position and nicely loosened up.

The knee kick is shown in illustration 27, f. The straight white arrow pointing upwards on my leg indicates the direction the knee kick has travelled.

Illustration 27, f. With the attacker all locked up, using my right knee. I knee kick him is the left side of his jaw.

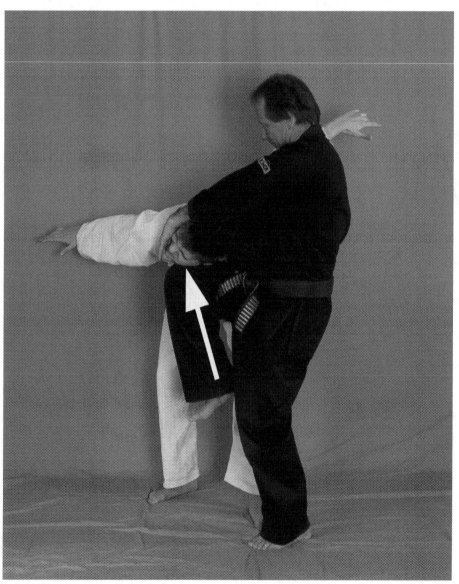

I am now ready to bring a conclusion to this rear strangulation and defence routine. I release my left hand from the attacker's chin and without putting my foot down, I stamp kick to the attacker's left foot with my right heel. While the attacker is "thinking" about this and all the other strikes, blows and locks I have applied since the onset of this attack, I am now able to make a safe exit from the attack area.

Illustration 27, g shows the attacker left foot being stamped on with my right heel stamping kick. The straight white arrow indicates the direction my right foot had travelled in to deliver the stamping kick.

Illustration 27, g. The rear strangulation and defence routine is concluded with a stamp kick to the attacker's left foot. Note: Adding a kiai to the stamp kick will give it more foot crunching power.

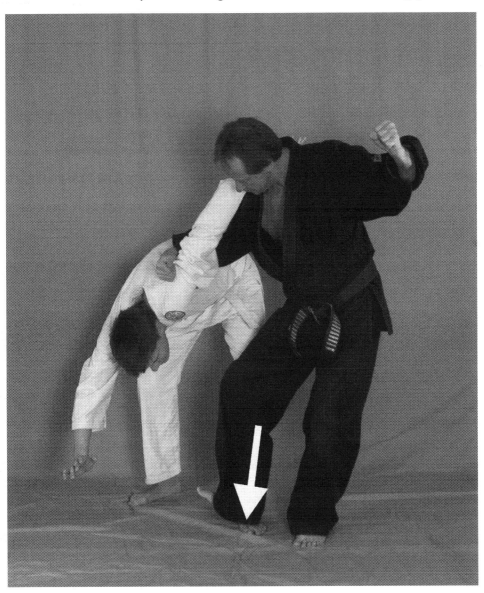

Ok, a bit of nagging, now that you have tried this routine one side, flip over and do it the other side.

Rear bear hug attack and defence routine into (三教 *sankyō*) a rotational wristlock. Ju-Jutsu style.

For the next attack, a rear bear hug, the attacker has been real crafty! He has managed to sneak up behind me and then grabbed me, restraining both my arms!

My immediate line of defence is not to panic. Then in two simultaneous actions:

1) I step back with my right leg, (this helps me regain my balance and also makes it a little uncomfortable for the attacker as it pushes him backwards.)

2) I raise both arms upward about fifteen degrees, this helps to limit the hold the attacker has on me by using the bodies own natural strength.

These action are shown in illustration 28, a. To help you follow these actions, the two white arrows by my hands indicate the raising of my arms and the straight white arrow on the floor indicates the step I took backward with my right leg.

Illustration 28, a. This attacker has grabbed me and is trying to restrain my arms from the rear.

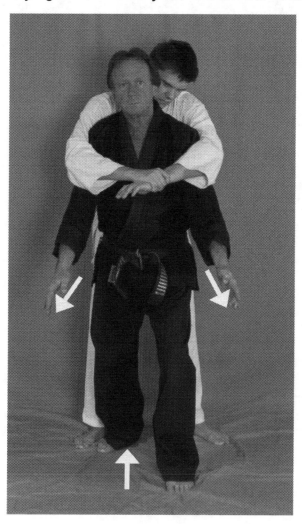

By raising my arms upward it has helped to create a small gap that enables me to grasp the attacker's right hand with my left hand. In this attack, the attacker has chosen to place his right hand on top of his left; this instantly dictates the hand I will take a hold of. If the attacker's hands were the opposite way around, then I would take at hold of his left hand.

As I grasp the attacker's right hand, I also extend my right arm out to my right side. This is the side I will exit from what I am doing at this stage is creating breathing space so that I can eventually duck under the attacker's right arm.

The above movements are shown in illustration 28, b. The small curved white arrow on my left hand indicates the direction that I have grasped a hold of the attacker's right hand in. The large white arrow on my right arm indicates that the arm is being extended.

Illustration 28, b. I take a hold of the attacker's right hand with my left and extend my right arm outward.

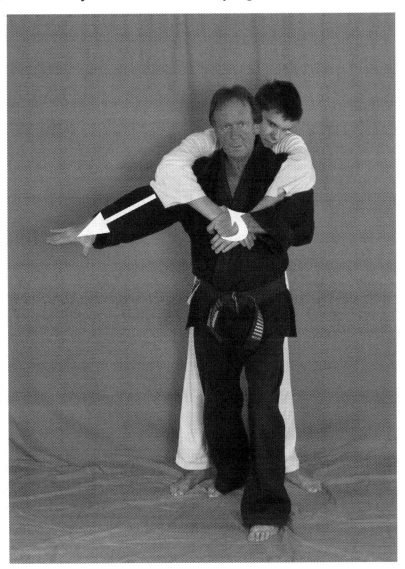

With the attacker's right hand secured by my left hand, I sight up the attacker left foot; then in a powerful downward action, I stamp kick it as hard as I can using the heel of my left foot.

As the stamp kick impacts onto the attacker's left foot, I instantly co-ordinate two movements together. My left hand starts to rotate the attacker's right hand clockwise; this starts to set up the wrist lock. At the same time, I elevate my right hand upwards; this raises the attacker's right arm up and creates more space for me to duck under it.

The golden rule for ducking under the attacker's arm is as follows: if you stamp on the attacker's left foot, you duck under the right or visa versa. The reason for this is; when you stamp on the attacker's left foot he automatically collapses into that direction; this makes ducking in the opposite direction easier.

The stamping kick and these two movements are shown in illustration 28, c with three added arrows to help guide you through the three movements.

Illustration 28, c. I stamp on the attackers left foot with my left foot, at the same time; I continue to set up the wrist lock.

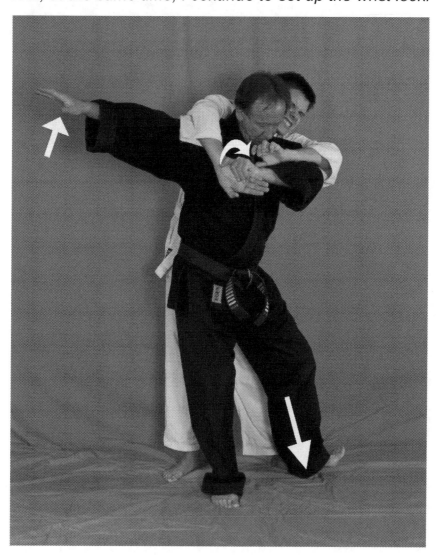

From the stamp kick, in one flowing action, I duck under the attacker's raised right arm, reversing my body to the attacker's right side. At the same time, I grasp the attacker's right hand with my right hand so that now both of my hands are now hold the attacker's right opened hand.

The positioning of each of my hands is important; the left hand is placed high on the attacker's hand, I have three fingers gripping into the fleshy part of the hand and one finger pointing, this finger is a "Ki" finger.....I will write a book on Ki one day and explain this, for the time being just point your finger. To stabilise the hand grip, the left thumb is placed just above the back of the attacker's right thumb. The right hand grips the attacker's fingers; again I grip with three fingers and point my "Ki" finger. To help you understand the intricate hand positions, I have included a small photo in the top left corner of illustration 28, d.

With my (三教 *sankyō*) in place, I turn the attacker's hand anti-clockwise; the (三教 *sankyō*) rotational wristlock is now applied. This is shown in illustration 28, d. The curved black arrow indicates the anti-clockwise rotation of the attacker's right wrist. The straight white arrow on the floor pointing to my right foot indicates my reversal to the attacker's right side.

Illustration 28, d. The technique (三教 sankyō) rotational
wristlock is being applied to the attacker.

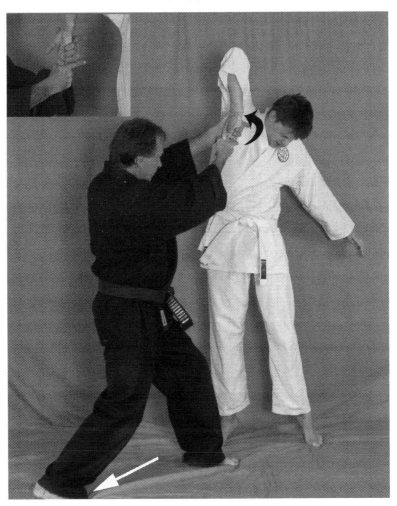

I maintain control of the rotational wristlock with both hands and then to further control the attacker, using the edge of my left foot (this is sometimes called the side blade kick, "ashi-gatana" or "sokuto" in Japanese) I deliver a powerful side kick (*yoko geri*) just above the attacker's right knee, this strike is another atemi point.

The side kick (*yoko geri*) into the attacker's right knee is shown in illustration 28, e. The straight white arrow on my left leg indicates the side kicks striking direction.

Illustration 28, e. Keeping the (三教 sankyō) rotational wristlock on, I side kick the attacker's knee.

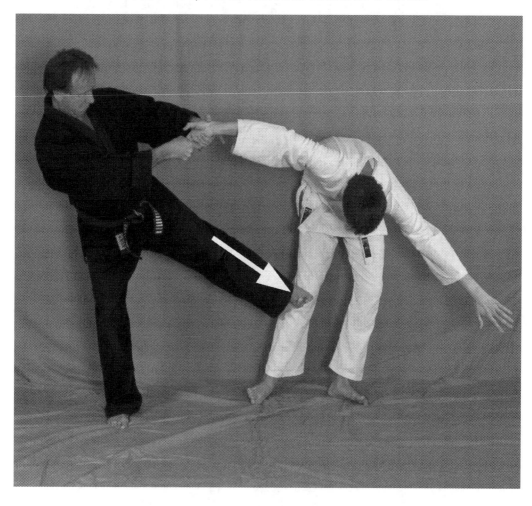

As the side kick (*yoko geri*) impacts just above the attacker's right knee, I release the (三教 *sankyō*) rotational wristlock and allow the attacker to collapse to the floor.

From the knee injury, the attacker has dropped to the floor, crouched down on his right knee and has his back exposed to me. I will now take full advantage of this prone position by finishing this routine with a powerful elbow strike (Empi or Enpi) into the centre of his back, this elbow strike is another atemi point. I have added a kiai for more power. The elbow strike is shown in illustration 28, f. The straight white arrow on my right arm indicates the direction the right elbow has travelled in order to deliver the elbow strike.

Illustration 28, f shows the conclusion to the rear bear hug attack and defence routine into (三教 sankyō) with a back breaking elbow strike.

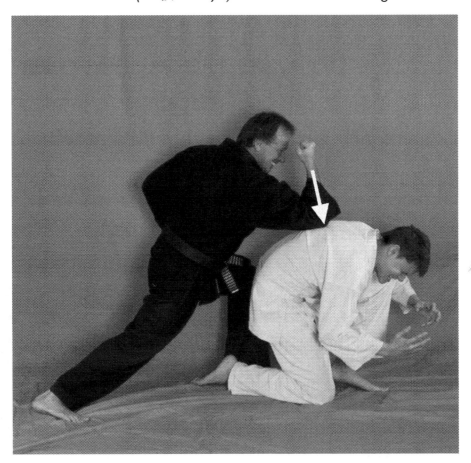

I know from a self defence point of view the rotational wristlock (三教 *sankyō*) is a complex technique. It is however a technique that is worth mastering, it allows you to restrain and control of an attacker whilst he or she is standing. More importantly, it gives you "fighting breathing space" when applying this technique to an attacker and using him or her as a human shield from other attacker's.

As you now realise the importance of this technique from a defensive tactical point of view, you will also understand the importance of practicing this rotational wristlock (三教 *sankyō*) both sides.

I have spoken about the street environment, the attack terrain and street awareness. To get a full understanding of these three important elements and how they work in Ju-Jutsu as an art for self defence and unarmed combat, the next range of defences will be done outside the Dojo environment.

Caution: If you wish to replicate these techniques, you and your training partners must be extremely careful! The Dojo has all the necessarily safety equipment for training.......the "street" a term I use for anywhere outside the dojo doesn't!

My defences from various attacks will now incorporate the natural surroundings of the attack terrain as well as the full range of Ju-Jutsu techniques. In using the natural surroundings to assist in my defences, the attacker will get more than he bargained for!

Hand on the shoulder and pull backwards down the stairs.

The first attack and defence routine is situated on a quite, narrow stair well. I have just turned the corner of a landing and am proceeding to climb to the top of the stairs. This is shown in illustration 29, a.

Illustration 29, a. I am alone on the stairs……..or am I?

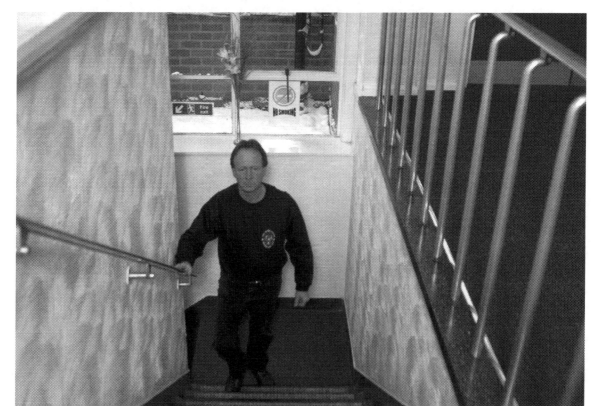

As I take the next step upwards, the attacker has sprinted up the stairs and has taken me by surprise by grabbing a hold of left shoulder with his right hand. His intention is to pull me backwards down the stairs; if I don't defend myself, then you can surmise that he will then beat the living daylights out of me, mug me and leave me for dead!

OK, I have painted a bad picture and am looking at the worse case scenario but, if you do not know what to do in this situation, who knows what the outcome could be?

The start of the stairs attack is shown in illustration 29, b. The attacker's right hand is on my left shoulder, the small white curved arrows indicates the direction the attacker is pulling in.

Illustration 29, b. The attacker has crept up the stairs behind me, grabbed my left shoulder and is attempting to pull me backwards down the stairs!

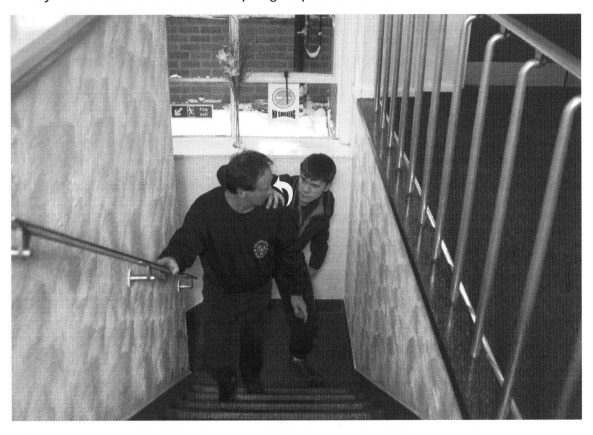

In self defence jargon, a shoulder pull back from the rear isn't a serious attack but, this attack is on a narrow stair well, where I am being pulled backwards down the stairs! My first problem is, the attack terrain; my feet are at different heights due to me climbing the stairs. The pull backwards immediately throws me off balance and I also have a chance of falling backwards down the stairs. This makes for a serious attack.

To stabilise my balance, I have to immediately co-ordinate two movements. Firstly, I instantly step backward down the stairs, leaving my right foot up one step and my left foot on the same level as the attacker. This has now stabilised my balance and I have a reasonable body posture. Secondly, using the natural street environment, my right hand keeps a grip of the banister rail, this also stabilises my balance and stops me falling backward.

With my balance stabilised, I am ready to fight back. In a powerful arc, I swing my left arm around and use my forearm to strike the attacker a stunning blow under the chin. As the forearm strike crashes under the attacker's chin he is knocked backward. This and the movements described to regain my balance are shown in illustration 29, c. The curved white arrow in this illustration indicates the direction that the forearm strike has travelled in.

Illustration 29, c. I step backward to regain my balance and then strike the attacker under the chin with a powerful forearm strike.

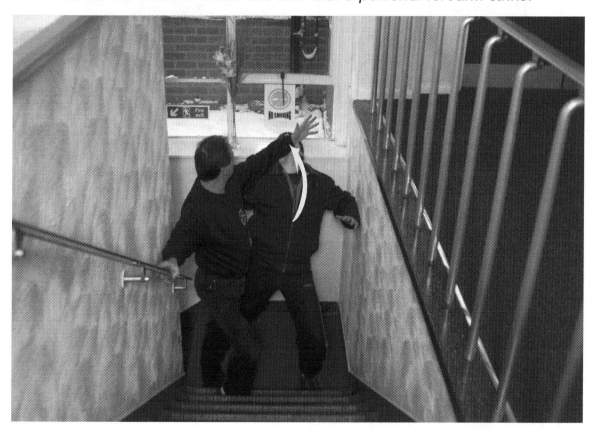

As the attacker falls backward from the forearm strike, I let go of the banister rail with my right hand, pivot my body 180 degrees (this positions me so I am now facing the attacker) and at the same time, using my right palm heel, I palm heel strike the attacker under his chin, this drives the back of the attacker's head into the window sill! This is shown in illustration 29, d. The straight white arrow on my right arm indicates the direction of the palm heel strike.

You may think that smashing the attacker's head into the window sill is an over kill but, the window sill is a natural part of the street environment. In practical self defence you have to be constantly switched on to your surrounding and what can be utilised in your personal defence. If you feel the street environment is alien to you, you will be defeated easily. On the other hand, if you feel secure with all terrains, street environments and have a high degree of Ju-Jutsu skills, you then have a good fighting chance of walking away from an attack and not being carried away in a body bag.

Illustration 29, d. Using my right palm heel, I smash the back of the attacker's head into the window sill.

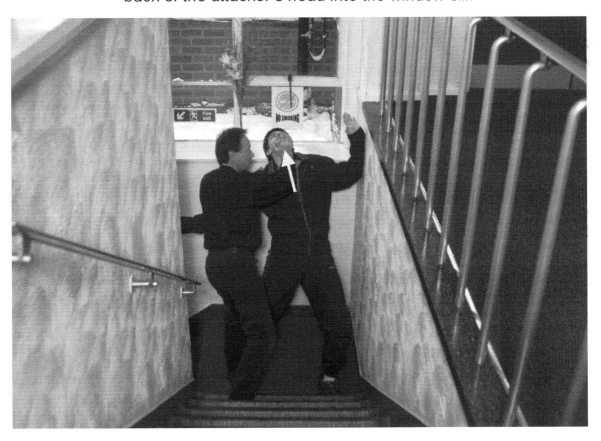

To conclude this self defence routine. I take full advantage of the attacker's vulnerable position with his head is back and his hips are forward, leaving his groin area wide open, using my right knee, I strike the attacker in the groin. With the attacker subdued, I can then make a safe exit.

The knee kick is shown in illustration 29, e. The straight white arrow on my right leg indicates the direction the knee kick has travelled in.

Illustration 29, e. The hand on the shoulder and pull backwards down the stairs is completed with a knee kick to the attacker's groin.

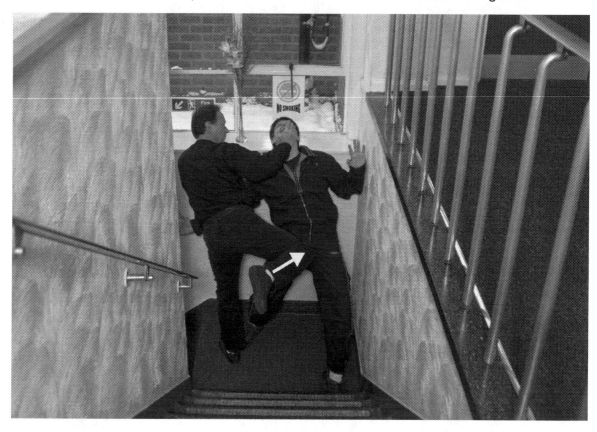

Defence from being smashed or pushed into a wall.

In the next attack, the attacker has with both hands grabbed a hold of my sweat shirt top and has tried to smash me into the wall. I emphasise......... try to smash me against the wall.

My first line of defence is to take a wall fighting stance. This stance is one that I developed some years ago and is perfect for all wall defences. The principle is simple; you use the wall to enhance your stance. Taking this stance will help reduce initial body impact and help protect your head and groin.

As the attacker tries to smash me against the wall, I instantly adopt the wall stance position.

1. Drive your back heel into the base of the wall.

2. Bring your opposite leg forward and drop into an hour glass stance. To explain the hour glass stance simply, turn both knees inward (this stabilises your posture and helps fend off knee kicks to the groin).

3. Arc your back so both shoulders are off the wall. If both of your shoulders are on the wall, the chances are that your head is also making contact with the wall......that's bad news! **Heads and walls don't mix!** So number

4. To avoid head injury, tilt your head forward to .

5. Breath out sharply as your body hits the wall; this will save you being winded.

Illustration 30, a, shows the attacker trying to smash me against a wall. I have adopted the wall fighting stance and have included two white arrows on the floor to help guide you through the foot work and hour glass stance. The other two black arrows indicate my shoulder and head are away from the wall. Please note, not shown in illustration 30, a; I have my hands up in a guard position.

Illustration 30, a. The attacker's initial attack, smashing me against a wall is foiled by me adopting a wall fighting stance.

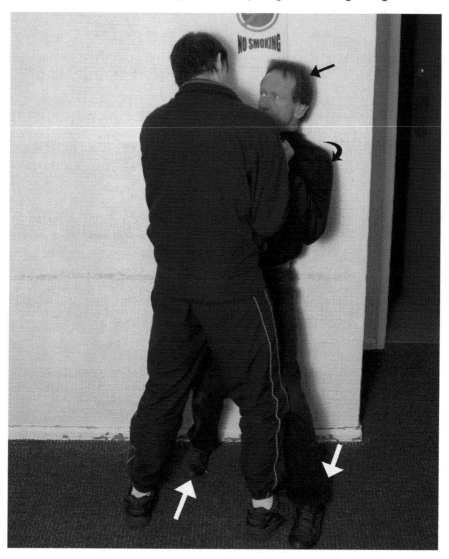

Once I have stabilised myself with the wall fighting stance, its time to begin my defence and escape strategy. To execute my first line of defence, I have to do three movements, step, draw and pull backward simultaneously.

From the hour glass stance, I extend my left leg forward; this is shown in illustration 30, b with a white straight arrow indicating the direction of the left step. The step shifts my body to the right side of the attacker. As I step forward, I hook my left hand into the bend of the attacker's right arm and draw outward. This drawing action is indicated in same illustration with a curved white arrow. In a simultaneous movement, I place my right hand on the attacker's right shoulder and pull backward. The straight white arrow in this illustration indicates the direction of the pull backward.

The combined efforts of all three movements now drive the attacker's head into the wall!

Illustration 30, b. The attackers head is driven into the wall.

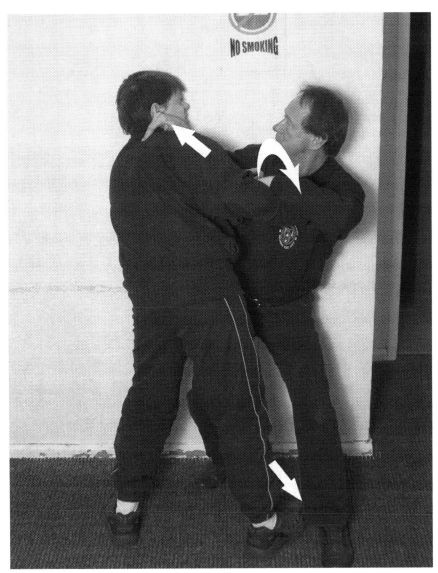

With the attacker stunned from his head being bashed into the wall, I give him another brain rattler, an elbow strike to the side of his head with my right elbow. At the same time, I grasp a hold of the attacker's right wrist with my left hand and then pull on the attackers arm to my left so it straightens out, (this procedure is setting up the next move).

These two movements are shown in illustration 30, c. The straight white arrow on my right arm indicates the direction of the elbow strike. The other straight white arrow on the attacker's right arm indicates that his arm is being pulled and straightened.

Illustration 30, c. The attacker's brain is being scrambled as I hit him with an elbow strike. At the same time, I am setting up an elbow lock by straightening out his right arm.

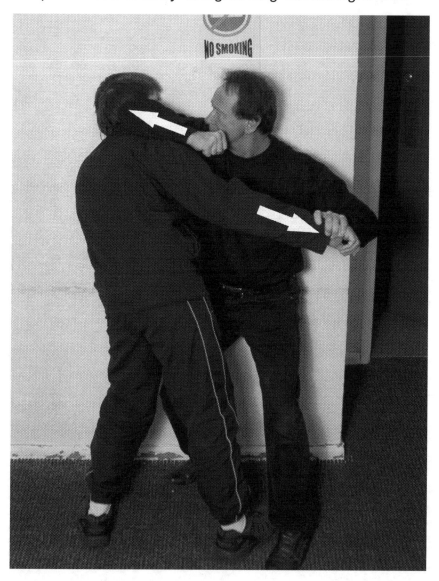

With the attacker now heavily subdued from two nice brain rattlers. I now wrap my right arm around the back of the attacker's right arm. At the same time, using my left hand, I rotate the attacker's right wrist outward, this helps align the attacker's elbow joint up for the elbow lock.

These movements are shown in illustration 30, d. The large white curved arrow in this illustration indicates the direction my right arm has travelled in and the small black curved arrow indicates the outward rotation of the attacker's right wrist.

Illustration 30,d. My right arm has wrapped around the back of the attacker's right arm in preparation for the elbow lock.

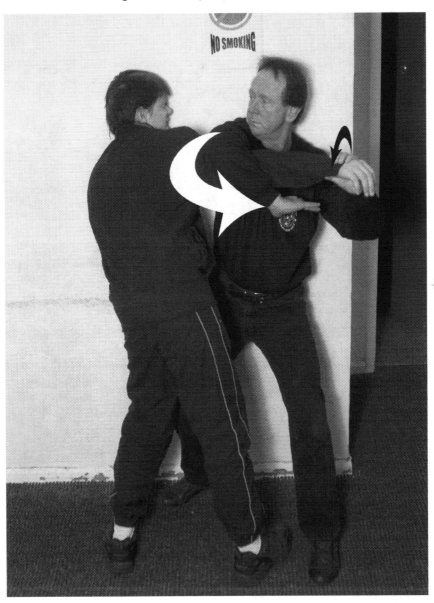

To apply the elbow lock, using my right hand I grasp a hold of my left forearm. I then push forward with my left hand and draw backward with my right arm. I now have a powerful **figure four elbow lock** on the attacker's right arm.

What also enhances this elbow lock is the fact the attacker is trapped face forward against the wall. As his body has no forward motion, the leverage power is immense, so when you practice this technique take it easy; it is incredibly easy to snap the elbow joint!

The figure four elbow lock is shown in illustration 30, e. The large curved white arrow in this illustration indicates the direction my right hand has travelled in to secure its place on my left forearm.

Illustration 30, e. The figure four elbow lock is being applied to the attacker's right elbow joint.

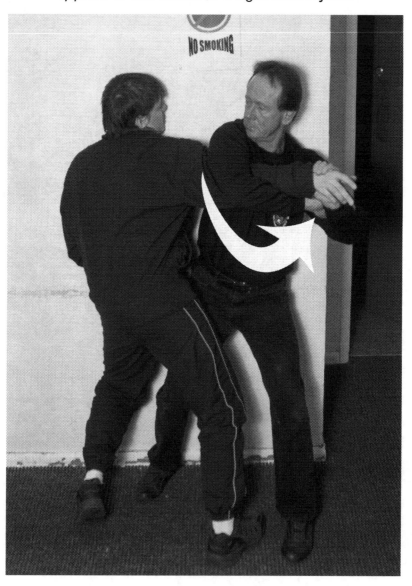

The figure four elbow lock is now used to help implement my safe escape and exit strategy. By drawing back as hard as I can with my right arm and pushing forward with my left hand, I use the leverage on the elbow lock to drive the attacker as hard as I can face forward into the wall.

With the attacker secured against the wall, I raise my right foot up and using my right heel, I stamp kick the back of the attackers' right knee. This stamp kick is shown in illustration 30, f. The straight white arrow indicates the direction my right foot has travelled in order to complete the stamp kick.

Illustration 30, f. I secure the attacker against the wall using the elbow lock. Then using my right heel stamp kick the back of the attacker's right knee.

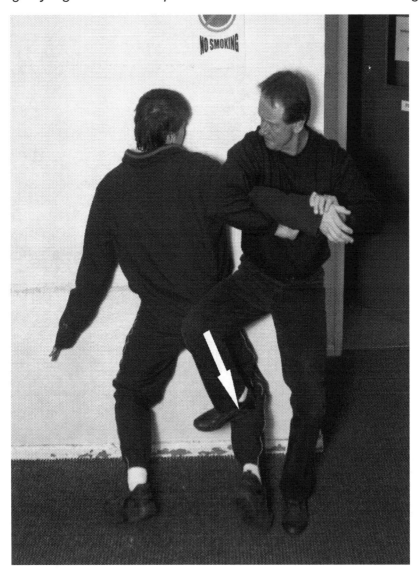

Now to conclude this defence routine and just to make doubly sure that I can exit safe and get no retaliation from this thug, who could be drugged, drunk, dangerous and crazy. I disengage the elbow lock and then using my right elbow, I elbow strike the attacker in the back of his head.

The elbow strike is shown in illustration 30, g. The straight white arrow indicates the direction the elbow strike has travelled in.

With the attacker reasonably subdued, I can now make a safe exit.

Illustration 30, g. To finalise this defence from being smashed or pushed into the wall. I do a final elbow strike to the back of the attacker's head before making a safe exit.

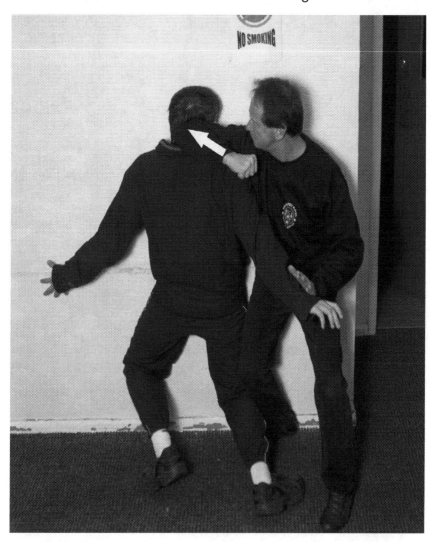

Seated attack with cosh or similar weapon.

In the next attack, the attacker has tried to take advantage of my seated position. He has used a simple ploy of asking me, the time? Can you spare some change? Or one of the million and one other devious ways thugs will use to get in close proximity to a potential victim. Once close enough, he has grabbed a hold of my sweat shirt top with his left hand. Then in a swift move, he has with his right hand pulled out a cosh that was hidden inside his jacket! His intention is to club me around the head with the weapon! If he is successful, who knows what will happen after that?

My first line of defence is to push my back into the chair and simultaneously extend my left leg out as wide as I can, this gives me a strong base and helps stop the attacker being able to push me backward off the chair. At the same time, I bring my hands up into a guard position. I am now in a chair fighting stance. This is shown in illustration 31, a. The large white arrow on the floor indicates the direction my left leg has taken in order to stabilise my chair stance.

Illustration 31, a. A chair fighting stance is my first line of defence when the attacker grabs a hold of me with one hand and produces a concealed weapon with the other.

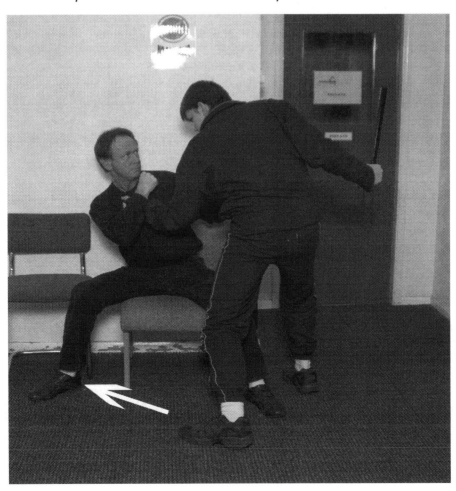

The attacker decides to make his next move, a vicious, right sided blow to the side of my skull!

My immediate reaction is to block the **attacker's right arm** (<u>not the actual weapon</u>) with a left outside forearm block. To enhance my chair fighting stance further, I have also pivoted on both feet; this dual action turns my body to face the attacker and puts me in a very low forward stance. Please note: The back of my left leg is still resting on the chair; this enhances the stability and power of my forward chair stance.

Illustration 31, b shows all of the above, as usual, I have added various arrows to help you follow the important movements. The large curved black arrow indicates the direction of the attacker's intended side blow. The large curved white arrow indicates the direction that my outside forearm block has travelled in. Finally, the two small curved white arrows at the back of my right and left foot indicate the pivoting action I have taken with my feet.

Illustration 31, b. The attacker swings a ferocious blow to the side of my head! However, his attack is foiled by me blocking it with a powerful outside forearm block.

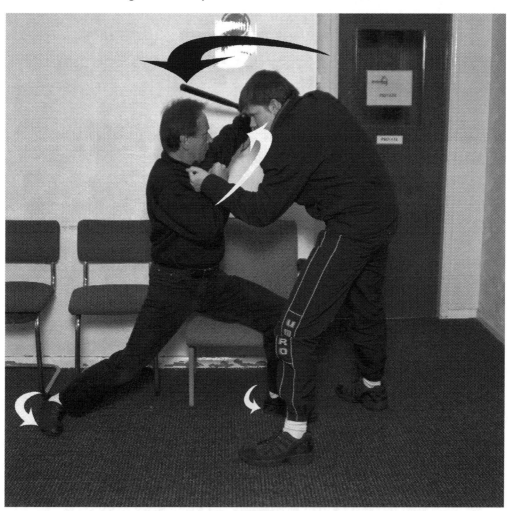

As you may have gathered, one of the key components to Ju-Jutsu is all about being able to execute multiple actions simultaneously. For the next part of my defence, I have to combine four movements.

Movement 1; I take a small outward step with my right leg. This takes my body off the chair and puts me in a low forward stance.

Movement 2; using the back of my right hand, I reach forward and flick strike the attacker in the groin.

Movement 3; as I reach forward with the flick strike the attacker's groin, I shift my head the attacker's right side. This stops the attacker head butting me as he reacts to the strike to the groin.

Movement 4; with my left hand, I grasp a hold of the attacker's right wrist. This secures his weapon arm and sets him up for the next move, a straight arm elbow lock.

Illustration 31, d shows movements 1 to 3. The small straight white arrow on the floor indicates the small step I took with my right foot. As you look at the illustration you will see a small curved arrow pointing to my right finger tips, this indicates the flick strike to the groin. The forth movement, the hand grasp is a little obscured but I am sure you will be able to follow this.

Illustration 31, d. With my right hand, I hit the attacker in the groin. At the same time, with my left hand, I grab a hold of his weapon arm.

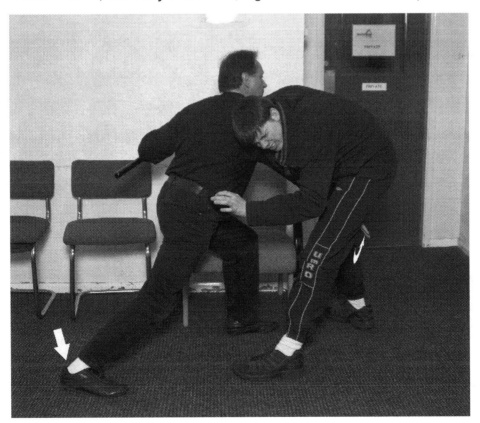

As soon as my left hand secures the attacker's right wrist, I move my right foot back to its original position; (this movement shifts my body to the right side of the attacker, it will help stop the attacker's upper body colliding with my body as I apply the elbow lock). At the same time, I elevate his right arm upward and then rotate his arm clockwise; this aligns his elbow joint correctly for the elbow lock. As a bonus, it also turns the weapon away from my head.

 Simultaneously, I hook my right hand just below the attacker's right elbow joint and draw forward in an anti-clockwise motion. These combined movements apply an extremely powerful elbow lock to the attacker's right elbow.

As the elbow lock is applied, it draws the attacker forward, transferring most of his body weight into his left front foot. This throws him off balance and stops any retaliation.

Illustration 31, e. shows the elbow lock being applied to the attacker's right arm. The small straight white arrow pointing to my right foot indicates the direction my right foot has travelled in. The other two small curved arrows indicate the clockwise (curved black arrow) and anti-clockwise (curved white arrow) movements used in order to apply the elbow lock.

Illustration 31, e. I raise the attacker's right arm upward and then apply a powerful elbow lock…or elbow break.

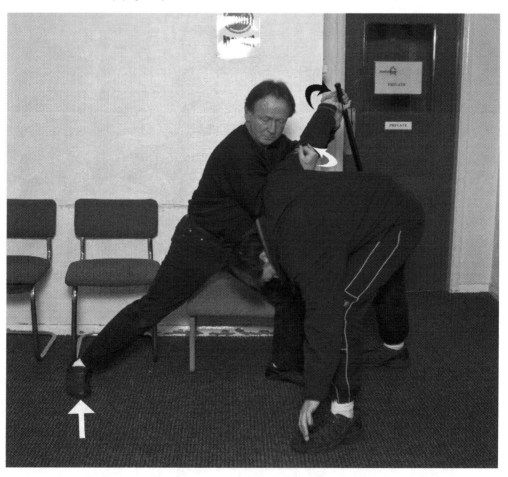

Now I need to disarm the attacker. From the elbow lock, in a smooth action, I fold the attacker's right arm up his back. As I do this, I aim his right hand towards my right shoulder; this puts a powerful shoulder lock on the attacker. It also brings the cosh he is holding into an easy disarm position.

While I still secure the shoulder lock with my left hand, I use my right hand and take a hold of the cosh's shaft and then prise it from the attacker's right hand. If the attacker offer's any resistance at this stage, I just put more pressure on to his shoulder by drawing his right hand closer to my right shoulder. Another option is: I can use verbal commands. In a strong voice I will tell the attacker **"LET GO OF THE WEAPON NOW"** If he does not comply then I will use the martial arts universal language, **PAIN.**

Illustration 31, f shows the shoulder lock being applied to the attacker's right shoulder. The large curved black arrow in this illustration indicates the direction the attacker's arm has travelled in from the elbow lock and into the shoulder lock.

Illustration 31, f. I am now able to disarm the attacker
after applying a controlling shoulder lock.

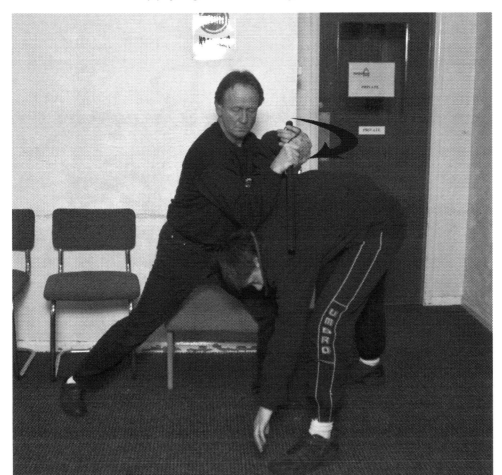

Now that I have control of the weapon, I want to exit the attack area safely. To do this I have to make sure that this lunatic who has just tried to smash my brains in with a weapon is unable to retaliate. You may be asking yourself why on earth would he want or even try to retaliate after all that I have done to him. The answer is simple, desperation.

When the attacker started his attack on me he was confident that he could pull this off and walk away with no fear of being caught. This is true of most armed and unarmed attacks. However the cards have turned on him, and in a few seconds, this little elderly man has turned his world upside down. He now faces being arrested and possible jail time, so now he is desperate to get away and that makes him even more dangerous!

To maintain control of the attacker, I keep the shoulder lock on with my left hand and draw forward so the attacker is kneeling on one knee. As the attacker is drawn forward his back is exposed to me. I then use my right elbow to strike a key atemi point in the centre of his back.

Illustration 31, g shows the attacker being controlled on one knee and the elbow strike to the atemi point being executed. The straight white arrow indicates the direction my right arm has travelled in to execute the elbow strike.

Illustration 31, g. The attacker has been pulled down on to one knee; the shoulder lock is still on him and has now been hit in the centre of his back with an elbow strike.

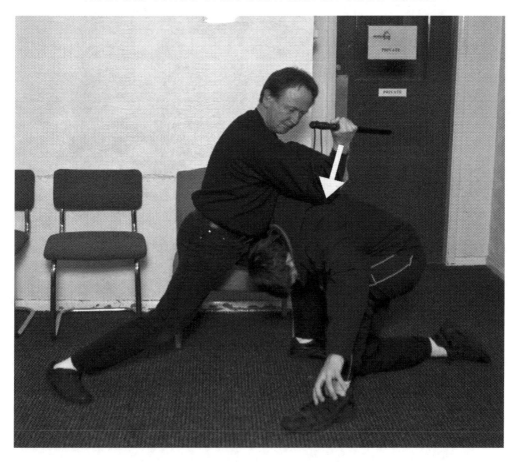

As I let go of the shoulder lock, the attacker makes one last desperate bid to fight back. However, his futile efforts are neutralised by a swift right knee kick into his jaw. In any attack situation, **always be prepared for fight back**, if it doesn't happen fine. If it does, its no big deal, you just deal with it. At the end of the day, it's all part of Ju-Jutsu training and becoming a good martial artist.

Illustration 31, h shows the completion of the seated attack with cosh and defence routine with a right knee kick crashing into the attacker's jaw. The straight white arrow indicates the direction the knee kick has travelled in.

With this done, I can now make a safe exit from the attack area. A safe exit entails the following:

1. Evaluating my own safety, an example is; check to see if any other potential attacker's are in the vicinity.

2. Taking control of the weapon and possibly putting it somewhere safe so it can't be used again.

3. Contacting the police and maybe the ambulance service..........for the attacker.

Illustration 31, h. The seated attack with cosh and defence routine is completed with a stunning conclusion. As the attacker attempts a final fight back, he gets a jaw breaking knee kick into the right side of his jaw!

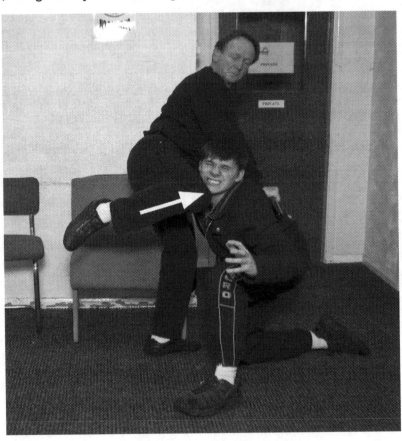

Knife across the throat attack, from a seated position.

The attacker has sat down beside me and engaged me in some harmless talk; this is to lull me into a false sense of security. All of a sudden, with his right hand, he pulls out a concealed knife and puts it across my throat! Then using his left hand, he grabs a hold of my sweat shirt top and pins me into the chair. The harmless talk is over; he tells me he is going to kill me if I don't hand over some money! This is an extremely dangerous situation, the fact is, it's happening and I have to deal with it. This initial attack is shown in illustration 32, a.

Illustration 32, a. From a seated position, the attacker has taken me by surprise by pulling a knife and putting the bladed edge across my throat. He will kill me if I don't give him some money!

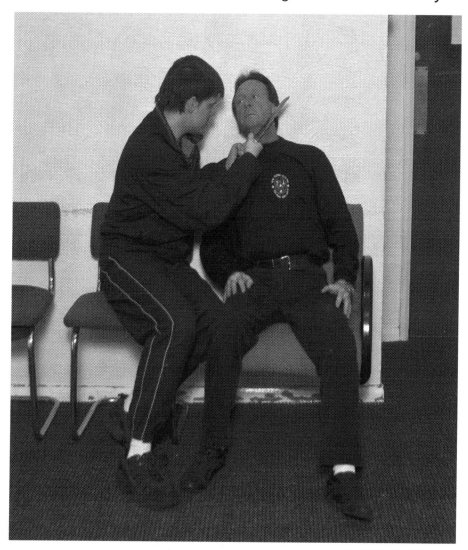

My first line of defence is to appear to go along with the attacker's demands. I inform him that I have a wallet in my right pocket with some money in it. I then ask his permission if it is ok to reach in and get the wallet. With his consent, using to right hand I reach into my right trouser pocket and get my wallet. I then offer the wallet to the attacker.

For the attacker to take a hold of the wallet, he has to let go of my sweat shirt with his left hand. This is just what I was hoping for. He has made his first mistake. His second mistake is a natural human reaction. When we are offered something our eyes automatically look at what is being offered. As soon as he takes a hold of the wallet and his eyes shift, I begin to make my initial move by cautiously raising to left hand. My intention is to grasp a hold of the attacker's right wrist.

Illustration 32, b shows the attacker has released his left hand grip of my sweat shirt top and is been given my wallet. It also shows with a straight white indicating the route, my left hand rising upward, about to take a hold of the attacker's right wrist.

Illustration 32, b. I hand over my wallet to the attacker. What the attacker hasn't yet realised is that this is part defence tactics.

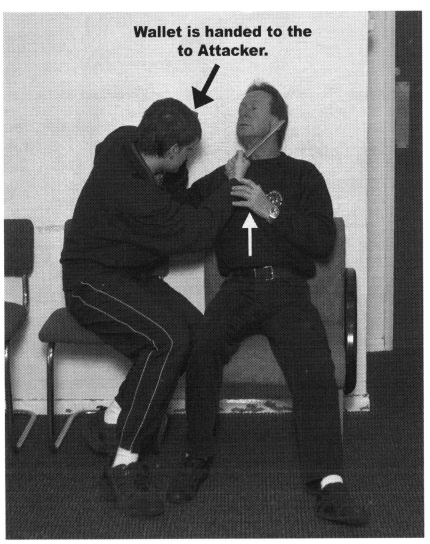

Wallet is handed to the to Attacker.

The next two moves are done simultaneously and with precision. Mistakes at this stage could cost me my life!

As the attacker takes the wallet from my right hand he believes he has made a successful mugging. I however view this differently; I know he has let my right hand get close to his face and I now take full advantage of this. With lightening speed and as much power as I can gather, I use my right fist and snap punch the attacker under his chin; this drives his head backwards and fractionally moves the knife blade away from my throat.

At the same time, my left hand grasps a hold of the attacker's right knife hand and I instantaneously rotate the attacker's wrist in an arc that directs the knife blade further away from my throat. This movement and the punch to the attacker's chin are shown in illustration 32, c. The straight white arrow on my right arm in this illustration indicates the direction the punch to the chin has taken. The small curved white arrow indicates the rotation I have made to the attacker's right wrist.

Illustration 32, c. As the attacker takes my wallet, I instantly snaps punch the attacker under the chin. At the same time, with my left hand, I rotate the attacker's knife hand away from my throat.

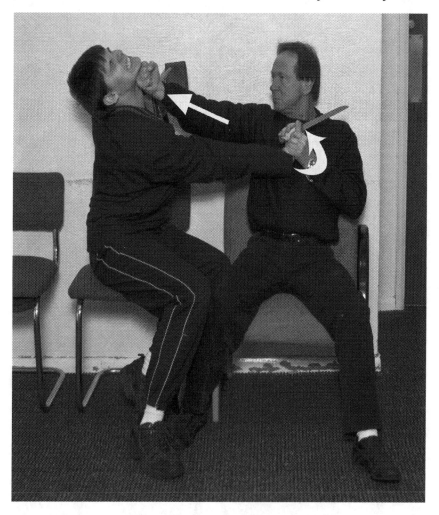

As the snap punch lands on the attacker's chin, I instantly stand up and reverse my right leg backwards. Please refer to illustration 32, d, this will show you the route my right leg has taken with an **L** shaped arrow the aid you further. The reason I have had to reverse my right foot in an L shape is that the leg of the chair is in my way and I have to step around it as I want to finally get into a strong stable stance.

As I step backwards, my right hand joins my left hand and they are now both placed at the back of the attacker's right hand. I then lever forward, this puts a wrist lock on the attacker and also puts me in control his weapon hand. Illustration 32, d shows the attacker's right wrist being locked up. I have also included a curved white arrow to help you understand the direction of leverage.

Illustration 32, d. From my seated position, I stand up and reverse away from the attacker. At the same time with both my hands, I apply a wrist lock to the attacker's knife hand.

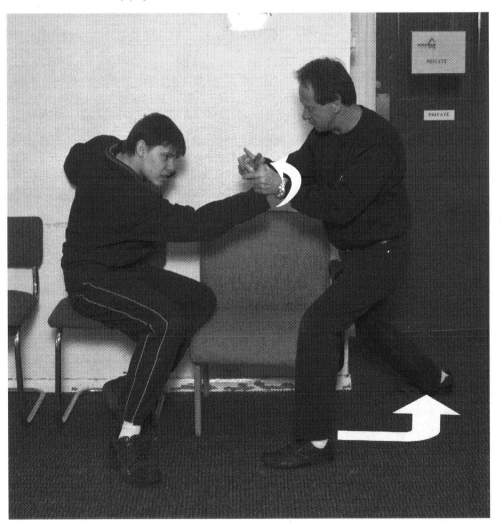

With as small adjustment, my right foot completes its journey and I am now in a strong stance. From this stance, I keep the forward leverage on the attacker's wrist and drive the attacker's knife hand downward so that the tip of his elbow smashes into the seat of the chair. The impact amplifies the wrist lock.........or should I say now, wrist break! Another bonus of these movements is that the attackers' upper torso is pulled forward and seated posture broken. This sets up the next move nicely.

These movements are shown in illustration 32, e. As you look at this illustration, the small straight white arrow pointing to my right foot indicates my foot adjustment. The small curved white arrow indicates the forward motion of leverage being applied to the attacker's right wrist. And finally, the other small straight white arrow pointing just above the bend in the attacker's right arm indicates the direction the attacker's elbow has travelled in as it crashes into the seat of the chair.

Illustration 32, e. While maintaining my grip and forward leverage of the attacker's knife hand, I smash the attackers elbow into the seat of the chair.

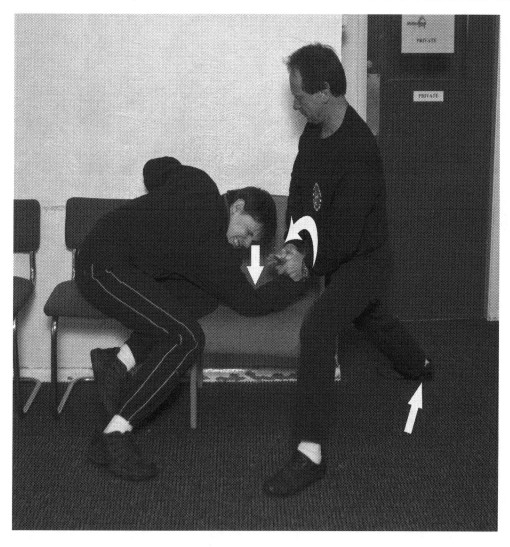

A badly injured or broken wrist will not stop an attacker from fighting back, especially if he has had a cocktail of drugs, alcohol and who knows what other chemicals he could have taken. With his system is in chemical overload, the brains pain receptors do not respond to pain until he comes down from his chemical high. I have to recognise this immediately and switch my defence tactics to an age old drug and alcohol counter method, wind him!

To do this, I keep the wrist lock on the attacker and his elbow secured to the chair seat with my left hand, this helps stop him from regaining his seated posture. Then with my free right arm, I bend my elbow, raise it high and then crash right into the centre of the attacker's shoulder blades. This is a stunning strike that knocks the wind right out of the attacker's lungs.....it also hurts like hell.........tomorrow this drug crazed son of a bXXXX is going to be in a world of pain!

The elbow strike is shown in illustration 32, f. The small straight white arrow on my right arm indicates the direction of the elbow strike. The small curved arrow indicates the wrist lock is still been applied to the attacker's right wrist.

Illustration 32, f. I maintain control of the attacker's knife hand; then using my right elbow, I knock the wind out of the attacker with a powerful elbow strike to the centre of his shoulder blades.

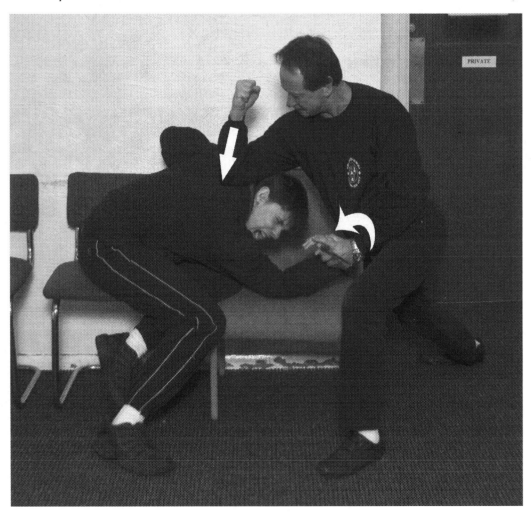

With the attacker stunned and gasping for air, it's time for me to plan my safe exit from the attack area. I keep the attacker restrained with the wrist lock and then remove the knife with my right hand. When I remove a knife from someone's hand, I always take a hold of the handle and withdraw it backwards; this makes it safe for me, if the attacker gets a little nick during this procedure, tough!

With the knife secured in my right hand, I again use my right hand and recover my wallet, this time from the attacker's left hand. This is shown in a very self explanatory illustration 32, g.

Illustration 32, g. While keeping control of the attacker's right wrist, I disarm the attacker and then retrieve my wallet.

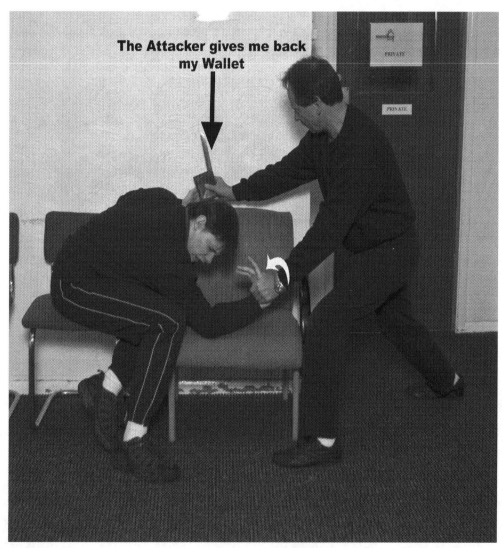

In life, some people never learn. As I let go of the attacker's right wrist, he decides to have one more go……the fool! From his seated position he tries to lung at me! Before he can blink, I fire out a front kick (mae geri) and the attacker's his chin collides with the ball of my right foot.

This final tooth shattering movement is shown in illustration 32, h. The illustration also shows that I have successfully taken control of the attacker's knife and retrieved my wallet. With that, I exit the area.

Illustration 32, h. The knife across the throat attack, from a seated position is concluded with a front kick to the attacker's chin. Once the kick lands, I make a safe exit from the attack area.

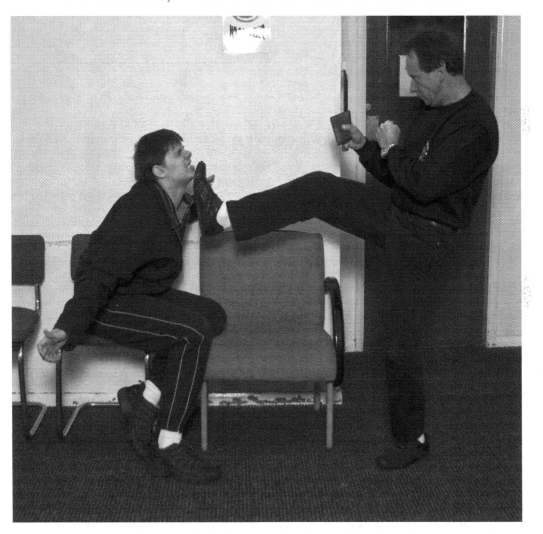

I know by now some readers will be asking "why don't you use the knife or whatever weapons the attacker has attacked me with on the attacker". The answer is; I abide by the law of the land. I am allowed by law to defend myself; this law says I can use reasonable force, this I have done. It does not make any allowance for me to go ballistic and kill or maim the attacker beyond that reasonable force. If I took it to level of using the weapon on the attacker: I would be arrested, taken to court and sent to jail for murder or if the attacker survives, grievous bodily harm.

Hand gun attack against the side of the head, in a seated position.

Any type of attack can be a traumatic experience. The next one is not just for the movies, it happening every single day, twenty four seven, not somewhere else in the world but right on your doorstep. A close quarter hand gun attack! Yes, this could happen to you and it's scary, but with the right techniques it is also defendable.

The attacker has been hiding behind the door at my left side, as I take a seat; he bursts through the door and shoves a hand gun in the left side of my head.

I realise that at this point of time the attacker in total control, he hasn't shot me yet so he must want something from me. My first line of defence is to do nothing to antagonise him; this means no sudden movements with my arms or legs. I keep still, eyes forward and wait for him to tell me what he wants. This is shown in illustration 33, a.

Illustration 33, a. Armed with a hand gun, the attacker has burst though the side door to my left and shoved the gun into the side of my head.

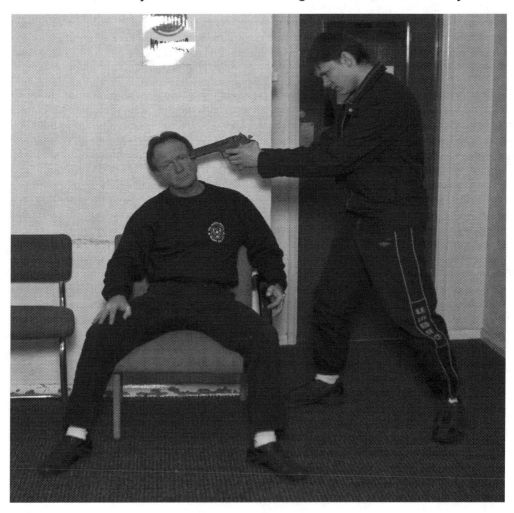

The attacker tells me to raise my hands; I do as I am told and act totally submissive. He then demands I give him some money. I inform him my money is kept in my wallet that is in my right trouser pocket and ask "is it ok to reach in and get it" With his approval, using my right hand, I reach in and take a hold of my wallet. This is shown in illustration 33, b.

The opening movements of any defence are always the most important ones, while what has transpired doesn't look anything yet, a few key things have already happened. My left hand is raised and is by the attacker's gun hand and the attacker has already taken one hand off the gun. Small as they maybe, these two movements are exactly what I want to happen and will ultimately lead to the attacker's downfall.

Illustration 33, b. The attacker makes his demands, he wants my money. I play his game to start with and in a compliant manner offer to hand it over to him.

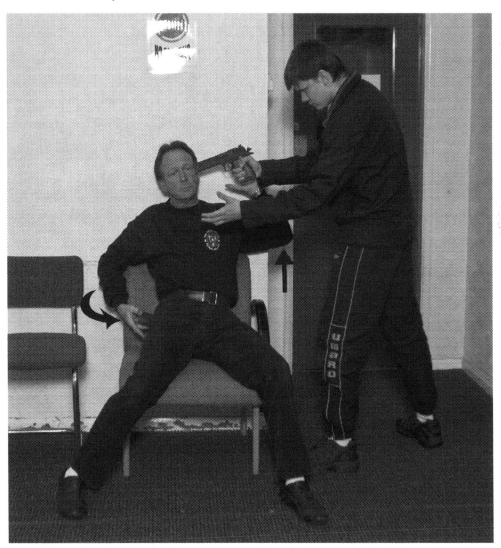

The next part of this defence is convincing the attacker that he is seconds away from a successful mugging. I therefore use my right hand and obediently hand my wallet over to the attacker. As I do this the attacker takes a hold of the wallet with his left hand. This is shown in illustration 33, c.

As you look at illustration 33, c it doesn't look like a great deal is going on; however it is a pinnacle point for both of us. So let's look at it first from the attacker's view point. He has just gripped the wallet with my money in it; he will now make a decisive decision as to what he will do next. Shoot me, pistol whip me and beat the living daylights out of me or let me go unharmed.

From my point of view, I have no idea what is going on in the attacker's head. At this point of time my evaluation is this is like a game of Russian roulette….with the odds stacked against me at two to one. These odds are not acceptable to me; I now have everything in place to make my next move to save my life, I have no option but to go for it.

Illustration 33, c. The attacker is about to take my wallet, but he may be in for a surprise.

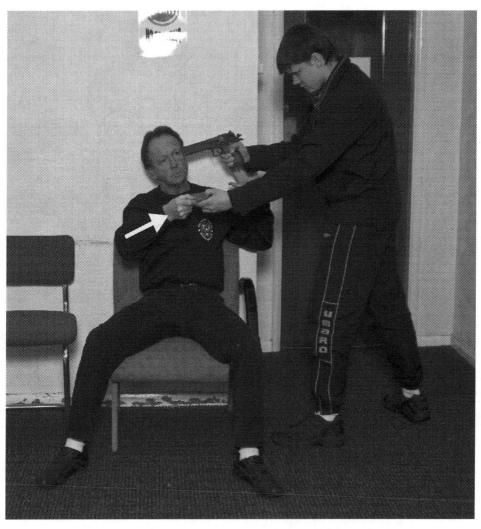

As soon as the attacker takes a hold of my wallet with his left hand, I grasp a hold of the attacker's gun arm with my left hand. Then in one powerful but smooth action, I drive the attacker's right arm upwards and slightly forward. As my upward driving action reaches a full arm extension, I rotate the attacker's arm outward. These actions takes about a millisecond, but in that time the attacker's gun has safely cleared my head and I have begun to set his right arm up for an elbow lock.

These movements are shown in illustration 33, d. The straight white arrow on my right forearm indicates the driving upward action of my right arm. The curved black arrow indicates the outward rotation I made with my right hand.

Illustration 33, d. In one fast action, with my right hand, I grab the attacker's gun arm and drive it upwards away from my head.

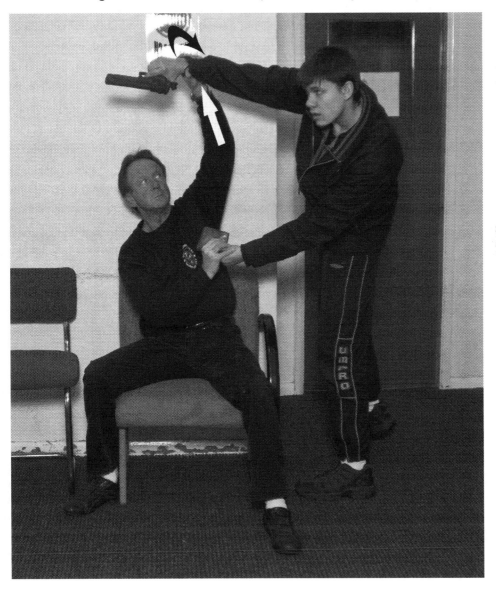

Using my left hand, I draw the attacker's right arm down and to my right side. As his posture lowers, I transfer the attacker right gun hand over to my right hand and immediately apply a wrist lock by bending his wrist upwards. This movement is shown in illustration 33, e. The small curved black arrow indicates the direction the attacker's wrist is being bent in order to apply the wrist lock.

It is only natural for the attacker to offer resistance to the wrist lock and also to try to regain his posture. To stop this and to apply an elbow lock, I place my left hand just above the attacker's right elbow joint. Then in two simultaneous movements, I push downward and rotate outward. This immediately applies an elbow lock; additionally the combined force of the elbow and wrist lock will restrict the attacker from regaining his posture. The elbow lock is shown in illustration 33, e. The small curved white arrow indicates the pushing down and outward rotational movements.

Illustration 33, e. The attacker is drawn off balance
and then a wrist and elbow lock is applied.

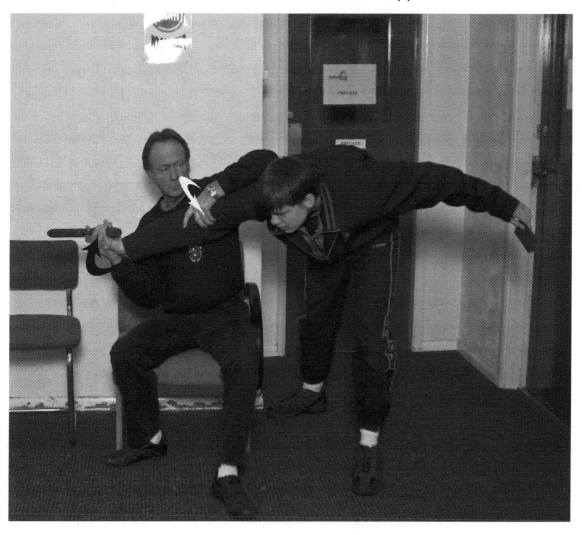

I keep the wrist lock on the attacker and also continue to drive downward with my left hand. These two locks being applied can easily break the joints they are being applied to. The attacker automatically goes into survival mode and collapses in order to reduce the pain. What the attacker hasn't anticipated is this only makes things worse! As his right knee hits the floor, from my seated position, I secure his right arm across my upper thighs. Now with his arm stabilised, I can apply more power into the locks! I also take advantage of his prone position by levering his right hand towards his right shoulder, this forces his right hand open and I am able to remove the gun from his right hand. Please note: for my own personal safety the gun is facing away from me as I disarm the attacker.

These movements are shown in illustration 33, f. The small straight white arrow in this illustration on the attacker's right leg indicates the attacker being forced down onto his right knee. The small curved arrow just above my left hand indicates the direction of force while applying the elbow lock. And finally, the small curved arrow by the attacker's and my right hand indicates the direction the attacker's wrist is being bent for the wrist lock and also the direction for disarming of the attacker.

Illustration 33, f. The attacker is driven into a kneeling position and while I am still sitting, I immobilise him with an elbow and wrist lock and then disarmed him.

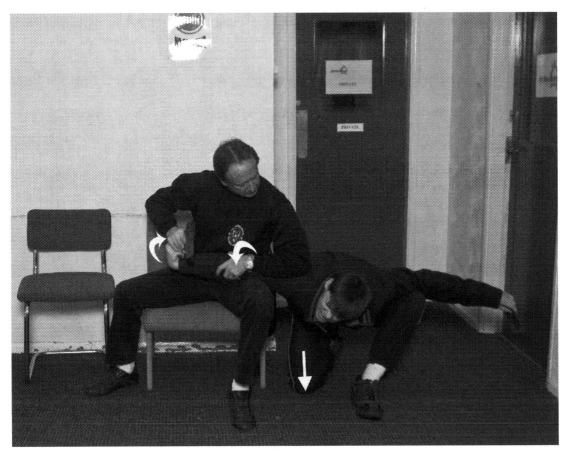

I am now at an important point in my defence routine, the fight back point. The attacker's elbow and wrist are locked and the attacker is feeling lots of pain and has lost control of the attack. Again out of desperation the attacker makes a wild attempt escape. But I am ready for this; Ju-Jutsu has taught me to expect this reaction. The attacker mentally blocks out the pain and tries with all his might to stand up. I do not oppose this; as he starts to raise his head, I release the elbow lock with my left hand and hook it around the attacker's chin and then pull sharply towards my left side, this pulls the attacker's back into the arm of the chair. This is shown in illustration 33, g. The curved black arrow indicates the direction my left hand has travelled in to grasp a hold of the attacker's chin.

Again I am doubling up on movements, at the same time as my right hand has removed the gun from the attacker's right hand, I use it to restrain the attacker's right wrist by bending it backwards and this action also helps maintain control of the attacker's right arm by keeping it drawn across my upper thighs. This is also shown in illustration 33, g.

Illustration 33, g. The attacker tries to fight back but I am one step ahead of him. As he tries to stand up my left hand instantly grasps his chin and I pull him backwards into the arm of the chair.

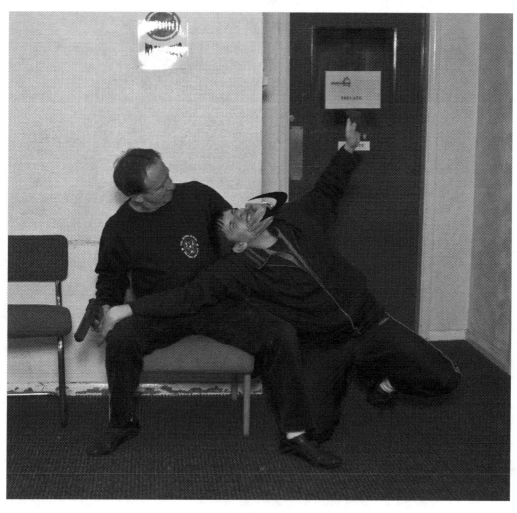

I continue to pull with my left hand until the attacker's back is arched over the arm of the chair and his head is tilting back as far as it will go. Then with the fingers and thumb of my right hand, in a vice like grip, I grasp a hold of the attacker's exposed wind pipe and squeeze. The result to the attacker is that his wind pipe is compressed and he is struggling for air. I know this is crude strangulation method but it works instantly and I have taken control of the attacker again. This is shown in illustration 33, h. The large curved arrow indicates the route the attacker's body has takes as he is pulled over the arm of the chair.

With the attacker secured by the throat grip, using my right hand, I point the gun at the attacker's upper torso. I do this for an important reason, safety. I do not know if the gun is real or if it has live rounds in it. Waving the gun around only puts others in danger! If it does fire accidentally then it will be the attacker who gets shot and not some innocent bystander. This is also shown in illustration 33, h.

Illustration 33, h. I haul the attacker over the arm of the chair, grasp his wind pipe with my left hand and apply a wind pipe throat strangulation.

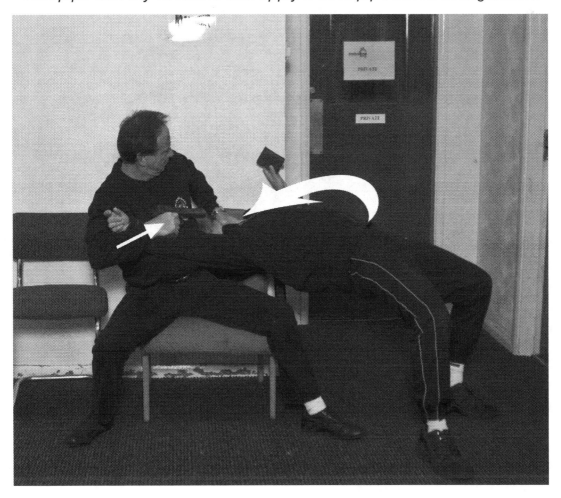

217

With the attacker disarmed and restrained with the wind pipe throat strangulation, I am ready to stand up. To maintain control of the attacker, my left had still keeps it grip on the attacker's wind pipe. I then slide myself off the chair and immediately take a deep forward stance by extending my left leg backward and my right leg forward, the right knee is bent to complete the stance. This is shown in illustration 33, i. The two small white arrows indicate the direction each of my legs has travelled in.

As soon as I am in my stance, I raise my right arm upwards, bend my elbow joint and then elbow strike the attacker in the solar plexus. The elbow strike is now ten times more powerful than a normal strike to this area. This is due to the fact that the attacker's upper torso is arched over the arm of the chair, this in turn pushes the solar plexus area forward and that makes the target area extra vulnerable to a strike. This is also shown in illustration 33, i. The small straight white arrow on my right arm indicates the direction of the elbow strike. Please note; the gun is pointing upwards for safety.

Illustration 33, i. I stand up, keep control of the attacker's throat with my left hand and then crash a stunning elbow strike into the attacker's solar plexus.

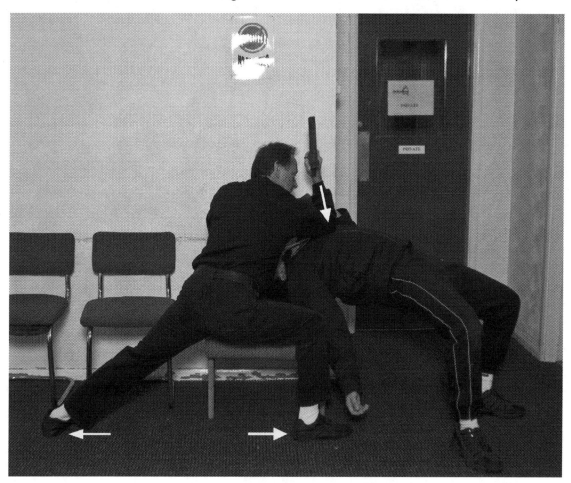

My defence from the hand gun attack against the side of the head, in a seated position is now complete; all I have to do in retrieve my wallet. Using my left hand I take the wallet from the attacker's left hand. This final movement is shown in illustration 33, J. Doesn't that picture look great, it looks as if the attacker's upper body is levitating over the chair!

Joking apart, before I exit the attack scene I have a few major decisions to make.

1. Is it safe to exit?

2. What do I do with the attacker?

3. What do I do with the gun?

4. At what point of time do I call the police? These are also the decisions you would have to make if you were in this type of attack and ones that I want you to take a few moments to answer. My answers to these questions are at the bottom of this page.

Illustration 33, j. I have successfully completed my defence from the hand gun against the side of my head. It is now time is take back my wallet and exit the attack scene.

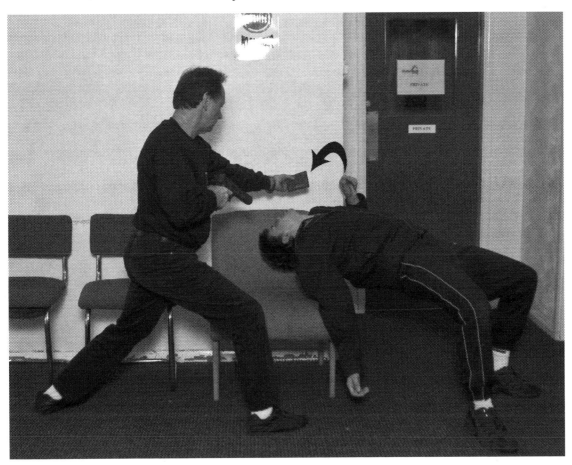

Answers to the previous questions, 1 to 4.

1. This confrontation has been one on one; it should be safe to leave the attack area as long as no other persons are threatening to attack me.

2. I will leave the attacker to sort himself out. I will not call an ambulance directly as I know I could be putting the ambulance team in serious jeopardy. I will advise the police that the attacker might need some medical assistance; they can then access the situation and implement a safe medical procedure.

3. I put the gun in a safe place immediately; I do not keep it trained on the attacker until the police arrive, they could on arrival interpret my actions as hostile and shoot me.

4. If any bystanders are around, I would ask if they have contacted the police, if not I would call the police as soon as I could; the person who has just attacked me needs to be locked away for a long time.

Mugging on the stairs, the attacker has a hand gun.

For my final defence for this book, I have linked the defence pictures together, this way you will be able to see instantly how I use Ju-Jutsu techniques and the natural street environment to defeat the attacker. The linked pictures from 1 to 6 are shown in illustration 34, a.

1. The attacker has been waiting at the top of the stairs for a new victim, me! He is armed with a hand gun and has it concealed from my view.

2. He points the gun at the side of my head and demands my wallet or cash, at this stage I comply.

3. I twist my body sideways and with my left hand I grasp a hold of the attacker's gun arm, this deflects the gun away from my head. At the same time, I take a step with my right leg and immediately punch the attacker in the groin with my right fist.

4. With my right hand I drive the attacker's right elbow into the metal banister railing, this applies an elbow lock.

5. I have swung the attacker's right arm from my left to my right and then using both hands I lock the attacker's right elbow joint on the metal banister railing, this draws the attacker's body over the banister rail.

6. I have passed my left hand behind the banister rail and then grasped hold of the attackers' right wrist; this locks the attacker's right arm around the actual banister railing.

Illustration 34, a. Hand gun mugging on the stairs. Pictures 1 to 6.

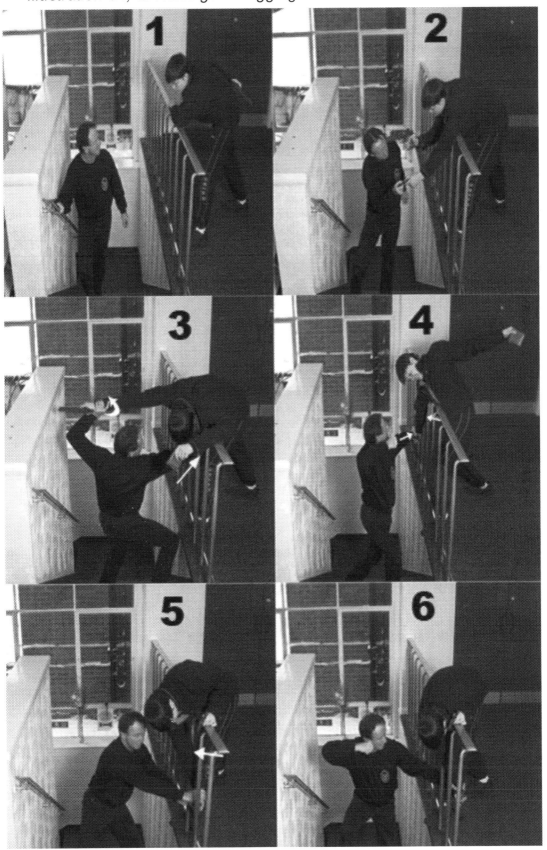

In picture **7**, I have added a curved white arrow to help you understand how the attacker's arm has been wrapped around the banister railing.

Picture **8** shows that I have taken a hold of the attacker's right arm with both my hands and am pulling his arm towards me; this will definitely break the attacker's arm! Picture **9** shows that using my left hand I maintain control of the attacker's right arm and have taken the gun off him with my right hand.

Picture **10** shows that I have move up the stairs and then using my right elbow, I elbow strike the attacker in the nape of his neck. As his head is resting on the banister rail, the strike should knock him out cold.

In picture **11**, I have retrieved my wallet and completed my stair mugging defence. All of the above is shown in illustration 34, b.

Illustration 34, b. Hand gun mugging on the stairs. Pictures 7 to 11.

Picture 11 shows the completion of this defence.

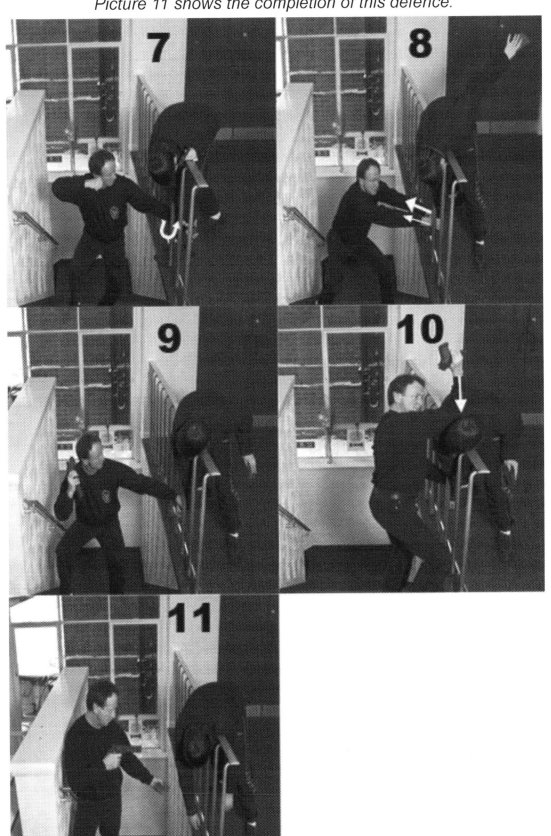

Conclusion of this book.

This now brings this book to a close; I sincerely hope that you have enjoyed the book and that some if not all of its contents will have been helpful to you in your study of Ju-Jutsu. Please remember Ju-Jutsu is a fantastic diverse martial art and this book has only scratched the surface of what you can learn.

In closing, I wish you well in your studies of the arts.

Best wishes, Sayonara

James Moclair

With Thanks

My thanks go to all my Uke's (Attacker's) for helping by patiently posing for pictures in this book; some of you deserve an Oscar for some of the great poses. Well done and many, many thanks.

A special thanks to Big Steve for all his help in proof reading the book.

Book trivia.

Time taken to write this book, just over one year, but it took forty five years of studying the art!

Words in this book over 56, 400

Spelling and grammar mistakes? You can add this one. Just remember the Author can't spell and was a poor English student at school, so please be forgiving.

Number of Pictures in this book 166. Ninety five percent were taken by James Moclair on a self timer.

All the pictures were personally edited by James Moclair.

The front and back cover was designed by James Moclair.

A

Abara: The ribs

Age: Rising

Age: Uke: Rising block

Ago: Jaw

Ago Uchi: A Strike to the Jaw

Ai Hanmi: Aikido Posture where both Exponents have the same Foot Forward

Aiki: Union of Energy. Harmony with Energy.

Aikido: A way of Harmony with **Ki.** Founded in 1920 by **Ueshiba Morihei**

Aikijutsu: Older Art of Aikido, Style Descended from the **Daito Ryu.**

Ashi: Leg, Foot

Ashi Garami: Leg Entanglement Technique

Ashi Guruma: Leg Wheel

Ashi: waza: Foot techniques

Atemi: A Strike to a Weak or Vital Point on the Body

Atemi Waza: Striking Techniques Used to Weak or Vital Points on the Body

B

Bajutsu: The art of Horse Riding

Batto: To Draw and Cut with a Blade

Bo: Wood Staff around 5' to 6' long

Bo-jutsu: The Art of using a **Bo**

Bogyo: Defence

Bokken: Wooden Sword, one that resembles a **Katana**

Boshi; Thumb

Bo Tanto: Wooden Training Knife

Bo Naginata: Wooden Polearm

Budo: Martial way

Budoka: A Person Studying Martial Arts

Bugei: Martial Art; the name for Comprehensive Classical Japanese Combative Systems

Bugeisha: A Practitioner of **Bugie**

Bujin: Warrior Person; Low Ranking **Samurai**

Bu-Jutsu: Catch All Term for all Japanese Martial Arts

Buki: Weapons

Buki-ho: Methods of using Weapons

Bunkai: Analysis of **Kata**. The True Meaning Behind the moves in **Karate Kata**

Bushi: Another word for **Samurai**

Bushido: The Way of the Samurai

C

Chi: Earth

Chiburi: Ritualized Shaking of Sword to Remove Blood

Choku tsuke: Straight Punch

Chuden: Mid Level

Chuden choku tsuki: Straight Punch to Middle of Body

D

Dachi: Stance

Daicho: Large Intestine

Dai: Large, Big

Dai Kinniku: Major Muscles

Dai Nippon Butokukai: An Martial Arts Organization First Established in 1895 in **Kyoto** Japan

Daisho: Pair Of Swords worn by the **Samurai.** A Long and a Short Sword.

Daitai: The thigh (also **momo**)

Dan: Rank; Denotes Black Belt Ranks. Ranks increase from 1 – 10.

De Ashi Harai: Advancing Foot Sweep.

Dembu: Buttocks

Denko: Atemi Point at the Floating Ribs.

Deshi: Student

Do: The Way.

Dojo: Place for Practicing an Art or Skill.

Dokko: Pressure Point behind the Ear.

E

Empi: Elbow

Empi Uchi: Elbow Strike

Empi Waza: Elbow Techniques.

Empi Uke: Elbow Block

Enga Osae: To pin face down

En Sho: Round Heel

Eri: Collar or Lapel.

Eri Dori: Lapel Grab

Eri Jime: A Strangulation Technique Using the Lapels

Eri Seoinage: A Judo Throw Done by Grabbing the Opponents Lapels

F

Fudo Dachi: Rooted Stance

Fuku Shidoin: Assistant Instructor

Fukushiki Kokyo: Abdominal Breathing.

Fukuto: Atemi Point just above the Knee.

Fumikomi Age uke: Rising Block Stepping In

Fumi Komi Geri: Stamping Kick

Fumikomi Shuto Uke: Knifehand Block Stepping In.

Fumikomi Ude Uke: Forearm Block Stepping In

Funakoshi Gichin: Founder of **Shotokan** Karate and Considered by Many to be the "Farther of Japanese Karate"

Futari Waza: Two Man Attacks

G

Gaiwan: Outer Edge of Arm.

Gaeshi: To Reverse

Ganmen: The Face

Ganseki Otoshi: Arm Bar with Elbow Brace Over Shoulder

Garami: To Entangle or Wrap

Garami Waza: Entangling Techniques

Gedan: Lower Level.

Gedan Barai: Sweeping Block

Gedan Choku Tsuke: Straight Punch to Groin.

Gedan Kake Uke: Downward Hooking Block.

Gedan Kekomi: Thrust Kick to Groin.

Gekon: Pressure Point to Lower Lip.

Gekyu: Low-level **Kyu,** the First Rank

Geri: Kick

Gi: Skill

Gi: Japanese Martial Art Uniform.

Gonosen-No-Kata; Judo, Kata of Counters

Go: Five

Godan: Fifth Dan. A Mid-High, Black Belt Rank.

Gokoku: Pressure Point in the Fleshy Area Between the Thumb and Forefinger.

Gyakon: Pressure Point on Lower Radial Nerve.

Gokyo: Aikido, Fifth Principle.

Goshi: Hip

Goshin Jutsu: Modern **Ju Jutsu** for Self Defence.

Gyaku: Reverse

Gyaku Geki: Counter Attack

Gyaku Juji Gamtame: Reverse Cross Arm Lock

Gyaku-Juji-Jime: Reverse Cross Strangle.

Gyaku kote gaeshi: Reverse Small Wrist Turn

Gyaku Tsuki: Reverse Punch

H

Ha: Tooth

Ha: Blade

Hachi: Eight

Hachi Dan: Eighth Dan

Hachimaki: Head Band

Hadaka: Naked, Bare

Hadaka Jime: Naked Neck Lock

Hai: Lungs (also Yes)

Haishu: Back Of the Hand

Haiwan: Back of the Forearm

Hajime: Start or Begin

Hakama: Divided Baggy Trouser worn while Practising Traditional Japanese Arts. They have Seven Pleats, Five at the Front and Two at the Back

Haito: Ridge Hand.

Haito Uchi: Ridge Hand Strike

Hanbo: 2-3 Foot staff.

Hanshi: Past-Master.

Hara: Stomach

Hara Kiri: Another term for **Seppuku** (ritual suicide.)

Harai: Sweeping

Harai Goshi: Sweeping Hip Throw.

Hariken or Hiraken: Fore-Knuckle Fist.

Hi: Spleen.

Hidari: Left

Hiji Ate: Elbow Strikes

Hima: Fore Head.

Hiza: Knee

Hiza Geri: Knee Kick

Hiza Garuma/Guruma: Knee Wheel.

Hombu: Head Office and Dojo.

I

I: Stomach

Iai: Sword Draw

Iaido: Modern Art of Swordsmanship.

Ichi: One

Ichiban: Number One, The Best

Idori: Techniques practised from **Seiza** (seated position)

Ifu: Dojo Tradition.

Ikkyo: Aikido Fist Principle

Ippon: Winning Point in **Judo** competition.

Ippon Ken: One Knuckle Fist.

Ippon Kumite: Practising Karate Movements using one Step.

Ippon Seio Nage: One arm Shoulder Throw.

Irimi: Entering

Irimi Nage: Enter Body Throw

J

Jigai: Japanese Women's Ritual Suicide Method.

Jin: Human/ Person.

Jintai: The Body.

Jin(zo): The Kidneys.

Jo: A Staff usually about 4 Feet Long.

Jo: Upper

Jo Jutsu: Stick Fighting Art

Jodan: Head Level.

Jodan Age Uke: Rising Block.

Jodan Tsuki: Upper Cut.

Jojutsu: The Art of using a Jo Staff.

Jonin: Ninja Leader.

Ju: Pliable, Ssupple and Yielding

Ju: Ten

Judo: The Gentle Way.

Judan: Tenth Dan

Ju Jutsu: Supple or Pliant Martial art. A Japanese Martial Art.

Juji: Cross.

Juji Gatame: Cross Arm Lock.

Juji Uke: Cross Block.

Ju-No-Kata: Judo Kata of Suppleness.

Jutsu: Art or Skill.

Jutte: Japanese weapon, Looks like half a Sai Dagger.

K

Kage Geri: Hooking Kick.

Kage Tsuki: Hooking Punch

Kaeshi-waza: Counter Techniques.

Kai: Association, Federation or Society.

Kaiken: A Short Dagger Carried by Women of the Bushi Class: Sometimes used to commit Ritual Suicide

Kaiten: To Spin, Turn or Spiral.

Kaiten Nage: Spiral Throw.

Ka-Jutsu: Fire or Explosive Techniques.

Kakato: Heel.

Kakato Geri: Heel Kick

Kama: A Smaller Version of Sickle.

Kamae: Posture.

Kan: House or Hall.

Kani Basami: Scissors Technique

Kano, Jigoro: Founder of Kodokan Judo.

Kansetsu Waza: Joint Manipulation Techniques.

Karate: Empty Hand

Kata: Shoulder

Kata: A Series of Martial Art Techniques to enhance the Art Practised.

Kata Guruma: Shoulder Wheel Throw.

Katame Waza: Grappling Techniques.

Katame No Kata: Kata of Ground Work Techniques.

Katana: Japanese Long Sword.

Katate: Single Hand.

Katate Yori: One Hand Holding other Persons Single Hand.

Katsu: The Art of Resuscitation also To Win, Be Victorious

Ke Age: Snap Kick.

Kekomi: Thrust kick.

Kempo: Iron Fist also known as Fist Law. Chinese Influenced Fighting Systems

Ken: Fist

Ken: Blade

Kendo: Modern Japanese Sporting Method using **Shinai** instead of Swords.

Kengo: Sword Master

Kenjutsu: Traditional Japanese Methods of using Swords.

Kenpo: See Kempo

Kenshutu: Swordsmanship.

Keppan: Blood Seal. A Vow or Oath Taken by a Student before being accepted into a Tradional School

Kesa Gatame: Scarf Hold

Ki: Inner Spirit or Strength.

Kiai: Unification of Energy: Usually Done by Means of a Loud Yell or Shout.

Kiai Jutsu: An Ancient Art that Concentrates on the Development and Accurate use of the **Kiai**

Kiba Dachi: Straddle Stance.

Kihon: Basics.

Kihon Kumite: Basic Sparring.

Kime No Kata: Kata of Self-defence.

Kin Geri: Groin Kick.

Ko: Minor.

Kodokan: The World Judo Headquarters Located in Tokyo

Kokyu: Breathing.

Koroshi: Death Blow.

Koppo Jutsu: Bone Breaking Techniques.

Ko Soto Gari: Minor Outer Reaping Throw.

Ko Shi: Ball of Foot.

Koshiki No Kata: Ancient Kata from **Judo**.

Kote Gaeshi: Small Wrist Turn.

Ko Uchi Gari: Minor Inner Reaping Throw.

Ku: Nine.

Kubi: Neck.

Kubu Nage: Neck Throw

Kuchi: Mouth.

Kuchibiru: Lips.

Kuzushi: To Break the Opponents Balance

Kyu: Boy

Kyu: Name Given to Grading System Building up to Black Belt.

Kyudo: Modern art of Japanese archery.

Kyu Jutsu: Classical Japanese Art Of archery.

M

Ma: Distance

Maai: Combat Engagement Distance

Mae: Front or Forward

Mae Geri: Front Kick

Mae Tobi Geri: Jumping Front Kick

Mae Ukemi: Front Breakfall

Maki: Wrapped around

Makikomi: Winding

Makiwara: Striking Board for Conditioning the Hands

Manriki Gusari: Chained Weapon with Weight on One or Both Ends

Matte: Stop

Mawashi: A Rotational Turn

Mawashi Geri: Round House Kick

Mawashi Tsuke: Round House Punch

Mawatte: Turn Around

Me: Eyes

Meijin: Someone who has Achieved Mental, Spiritual, and Physical Perfection in their Art

Men: Head, Face

Migi: Right

Migi Suki Geri: Crescent Kick

Mimi: Ears

Momo: Thigh

Mon: Japanese Crest

Morote: Using both Hands

Morote Gyaku Soto Uke: Reinforced Reversed Outside Forearm Block

Morote Gyaku Tsuki: Reinforced Reverse Punch

Morote Jodan Age Uke: Reinforced Rising Block

Morote Koken Uchi: Reinforced Arc Fist Strike

Morote Nukite Uchi: Reinforced Straight Finger Strike

Morote Shuto Uchi: Reinforced Knife Edge Hand Strike

Morote Sote Uke: Reinforced Outside Forearm Block

Mune: Chest

Mushin: State of Mind when Facing an Opponent. The Mind should be Clear of Thought

N

Nagashi: Flowing

Nagashi Waza: Flowing Techniques

Nage: Throw

Nage Waza: Throwing Technique

Naginata: Polearm Weapon with Long Shaft and Curved Blade

Naifu: Knife

Naka: Centre or Middle

Nakadaka: Middle Knuckle

Nami Jiji Jime: Normal Cross Strangle

Neko Ashi Dachi: Cat Stance

Ni: Two

Nidan: Second Dan

Nihon also Nippon: The correct Name for Japan

Nihon Nukite: Two Finger strike

Nikkyo: Aikido Second Principle

Ninja: Japanese Assassin, Spy

Ninja-To: Ninja Sword, Straight Blade

Ninjutsu: The Art of Stealth

Ninpo: The Ninja Way

Nodo: Throat

Nukite: Straight Fingers Spear Hand

Nunchaku: Rice Flail, Two Sticks made from various materials attached by a cord or chain

O

O: Great, Major

O Goshi: Major Hip Throw

O Guruma: major Wheel

O Soto Gari: Major Outer Reaping Throw

O Uchi Gari: Major Inner Reaping Throw

Obi: Belt

Obi Otoshi: Belt Lifting Drop

Okuden: Secret Techniques

Okuri Eri Jime: Sliding Collar Neck Lock

Osae: Immobilize

Osae Komi: Called in Judo Competitions to Recognize a Hold Down

Osae Waza: Immobilization Techniques

O Sensei: Great Teacher

P

Pinan: A Group of Five Basic Okinawan Kata's

R

Randori: Free Style Sparring

Rei: Bow

Reigi: Etiquette

Renshu: Hard Work

Renzoku: Geri: Combination Techniques

Ritsu Rei: Standing Bow

Roku: Six

Rokodan: Sixth Dan

Ronin: Samurai Warrior. With no Lord

Ryote Dori: Holding Both Hands

Ryu: An Art, Style

S

Sabaki: Body Motion

Sai: A Steel Trident

Samurai: Ancient Japanese Warrior. One Who Serves

San: Three

Sanchin Dachi: Hour Glass Stance

Sandan: Third Dan

Sankyo: Aikido Third Principle

Saya: Scabbard

Seika Tanden: Lower Abdomen. The Seat of Energy Based Three Inches Below the Navel

Seiken: Forefist

Seiken Tsuke: Forefist Strike

Seikichu: The Spine

Seionage: Shoulder Throw

Semban Nage: Shuriken Throwing Techniques

Sempai: Senior Student

Sen: The Number 1000

Senaka: The Back of the Body

Senjutsu: Tactics

Sensei: Teacher or Instructor

Sensei Ni Rei: Bow to the Teacher

Seppuka: Japanese Ritual Suicide

Shi: Four

Shiatsu: Tem for Japanese Acupressure Massage

Shichi: Seven

Shihan: A Senior Instructor

Shiho: Four Directions

Shiho Nage: Four Direction Throw

Shin: Heart

Shinai: Bamboo Sword used in **Kendo**

Shintai: The Body

Shomen: Face, Front Head

Shomen Uchi: Downward Blow

Shougun: General

Shuriken: Throwing Stars

Shuto: Knife Edge Hand

Shuto Uchi: Knife Edge Hand Strike

Shuto Uke: Knife Edge Hand Block

Sode: Sleeve

Sode Dori: Sleeve Grab

Sode Tsuri Komi Goshi: Sleeve Lift Pull Hip Throw

Soji: The Cleaning of the **Dojo**

Sojutsu: Spear Art

Soke: Head of Family and Head of Style

Sokei: Groin

Sokuso: Tips of the Toes

Sokutei: Bottom of the Heel

Sokuto: Edge of the Foot

Sokuto Yoko Geri: Side Kick Using the Edge of the Foot

Soto: Outer, Outside

Soto Uke: Outside Forearm Block

Suigetsu: Solar Plexus

Sukui: Scooping

Sukui Uke: Scooping Block

Sumi Gaeshi: Corner Throw

Sutemi Waza: Sacrifice Throw

Suwatte: Sit Down

T

Tabi: Shoes and Socks Divided by the Big Toe

Tachi: Standing

Tachi: Battle Sword longer than a **Katana**

Tachi Waza: Standing Techniques

Tai: Body

Tai Jutsu: Body Art, Skill. Old **Ju-Jutsu** System

Tai Otoshi: Body Drop

Taisabaki: Evasive Body Movement Using Circular Movement with the Feet

Tameshiwari: Showing Skill and Power by Demonstrating Breaking Techniques

Tan: Gallbladder

Tanden: Abdomen

Tani: Valley

Tani Otoshi: Valley Drop

Tanko: Bladder

Tanto: Knife with a blade between 4" and 13" The Knife used in Ritual Suicide

Tanto Jutsu: knife Fighting Skills

Tatami: Mat Area

Tate Shiho Gatame: Vertical four Quarters Hold

Tawara Geashi: Bale Throw

Teisho: Palm Heel on the Hand

Teisho Uke: Palm heel Block

Tem Ben Nage: Elbow Lock Throw

Tenchi: Heaven and Earth

Tenchi Nage: Heaven and Earth Throw

Tenkan: The Opposite to **Irimi.** To Go to the Outside

Tettsui: Hammer Fist

Te Waza: Hand Techniques

Tobi: Jump

Tobi Geri: Jumping Kick

Token Jutsu: Blade Throwing Techniques

Tonfa: Wood Staff with a Handle on the Side

Tori: Defender

Tsuki: punch

Tsuke Waza: Punching Techniques

U

Uchi: Strike

Uchi Waza: Striking techniques

Ude: The Arm. Inside

Ude Garame: Entangled Arm Lock

Ude Gatame: Arm lock with Hands

Ude Uke: Inside Forearm Block

Uke: Attacker

Ukemi: Breakfalls

Uki: Floating

Uki Goshi: Floating Hip Throw

Ura: Back

Ura Nage: Back Throw

Uraken: Back of the Fist

Uraken Uchi: Backfist Strike

Ushiro: Rear, Behind

Ushiro Geri: Back Kick

Uwagi: Uniform Jacket

W

Wake Gatami: Elbow Lock

Waki: Side: Armpit

Wan: Arm

Wanto: Arm Sword

Wakizashi: A Short Sword Carried as a Companion to the **Katana**

Waza: Technique

Y

Yama: Mountain

Yame: Stop

Yari: Spear

Yari Jutsu: Spear Throwing Techniques

Yoi: Ready

Yoko: To the Side

Yoko Geri: Side Kick

Yoko Guruma: Side Wheel Throw

Yoko Uchi: A Side Strike

Yoko Ukemi: Side Breakfall

Yokomen: Side of the Head

Yokomen Uchi: A Blow to the Side of the Head

Yonkyo: Aikido Fourth Principle

Yoroi: Armor

Toroi Nage: Armor Throws

Yowai: Weak

Yowaki: Weak Energy

Yubi: Finger

Yudansha: Black Belt Level

Yuki: Courage

Yukuri: Slow

Yumi: A Bow as used in **Kyudo**

Z

Za: Sitting

Za Rei: Kneeling Salutation (Bow)

Zanshin: State of Awareness

Zekken: Badge with ones own name or the Dojo Name on it

Zen: Philosophy and a Religion

Zenkutsu Dachi: Forward Stance

Zori: Japanese Sandals for use off the **Tatami** in the Dojo

Zubon: Trousers

Japanese Terminology phonetically broken down.

It can be daunting to try to learn a martial art and it is even more frustrating to try to pick up some of the terminology that goes with this, so the terminology has been broken down to help you pronounce it. Good luck!

Aiki Jutsu Terms

Shiho Nage (she-ho na-gay) - Four Directional Throw

Kote Gaeshi (ko-tey guy-ash-ee) - Small Wrist Turn

Irimi Nage (ee-ree-me na-gay) - Enter Body Throw

Kaiten Nage (kite-en na-gay) - Spiral Throw

Tenchi Nage (ten-chee na-gay) - Heaven and Earth Throw

Ikkyo (ee-key-o) - First Principle.

Nikkyo (knee-key-o) - Second Principle.

Sankyo (san-key-o) - Third Principle.

Yonkyo (yon-key-o) - Fourth Principle

Irimi (ee-ree-me) – Positive (inside or to enter)

Tenkan (ten-can)– Negative (outside or to not enter)

Judo Terms

O-Goshi (o go-she) – Major Hip Throw

O-Soto-Gari (o so-toe ga-ree) – Major Outer Reaping Throw

Tai-Otoshi (tie o-toe-she) – Body Drop

Ippon-Sieo-Nage (ip-on sea-o na-gay) – One Armed Shoulder Throw

Tsuri-Komi-ashi (sue-ree ko-mee ash-ee) – Drawing Ankle Throw

Kubi-Nage (ku-bee na-gay) – Neck Throw

Kesa-Gatame (kay-sa ga-ta-may) – Scarf Hold

Kata-Gatame (ka-ta ga-ta-may) – Shoulder Hold

Yoko-Shiho-Gatame (yo-ko she-ho ga-ta-may) – Side Four Quarters Hold

Tate-Shiho-Gatame (tat-ay she-ho ga-ta-may) – Vertical Four Quarters Hold

Kami-Shiho-Gatame (kar-mee she-ho ga-ta-may) – Upper Four Quarters Hold

Juji-Gatame (ju-jee ga-ta-may) – Cross Arm Lock

Okuri-Eri-Jime (o-kew-ree er-ee gee-me) – Sliding Collar Neck Lock

Kata-Ha-Jime (ka-ta ha gee-me) – Single Wing Choke

Hadka-Jime (ha-da-ka gee-me) – Naked Neck Lock

Uke Goshi (oo-key go-she) – Floating Hip Throw

Kime No Kata Terms

Kneeling – Idori (ee-do-ree)

Ryote-Dori (ri-o-toe do-ree) – Hold With Both Hands

Tsukkake (sue-k-ay-key) – Blow With Fist To Stomach

Suri-Age (sue-ree ag-ee) – Glancing Blow To Face

Yoko-Uchi (yo-ko oo-chee) – Blow From Side

Usihro-Dori (you-she-row do-or-ee) – Hold On Shoulders From Behind/Side

Tsukkomi (sue-k-o-mee) – Thrust With Knife To Stomach

Kiri-Komi (key-ri ko-me) – Cleave To Head With Knife (cut to head with blade of knife)

Yoko-Tsuki (yo-ko sue-key) – Axe Pick From Side

Standing – Tachi (ta-chee)

Ryote-Dori (ri-o-toe do-ree) – Hold With Both Hands

Sode-Tori (so-day toe-ree) – Hold On Sleeve

Tsukkake (sue-k-ay-key) – Blow With Fist To Stomach

Tsuki-Age (sue-key ag-ee) – Blow To Face

Suri-Age (sue-ree ag-ee) – Glancing Blow To Face

Yoko-Uchi (yo-ko oo-chi) – Blow From Side

Ke-Age (key ag-ee) – Kick to Lower Abdomen

Usihro-Dori (you-she-row do-or-ee) – Hold On Shoulders From Behind/Side

Tsukkomi (sue-k-o-mee)– Thrust With Knife To Stomach

Kiri-Komi (key-ree ko-mee) – Cleave to Head with Knife (cut to head with blade of knife)

Nuke-Kake (new-key kay-key – Block Sword in Sheath

Kiri-Oroshi (key-ri o-ro-she) – To Cleave With Sword

Karate Terms

JODAN AGE UKE (jo-dan ag-ee oo-key)	RISING BLOCK
GEDAN BARAI (gay-dan bar-ree)	DOWNWARD BLOCK
UDE UKE (oo-day oo-key)	INSIDE FOREARM BLOCK
SOTO UKE (so-toe oo-key)	OUTSIDE FOREARM BLOCK
GYAKU SOTO UKE (guy-a-ku so-toe oo-key)	REVERSE OUTSIDE FOREARM BLOCK
ZENKUTSU DACHI (zen-koot-sue ta-chi)	FRONT STANCE
JU DACHI (jew ta-chi)	FREESTYLE FIGHTING STANCE
KIBA DACHI (key-ba ta-chi)	STRADDLE STANCE
OIE TSUKI (oi sue-key)	LUNGE PUNCH
GYAKU TSUKI (guy-a-ku sue-key)	REVERSE PUNCH
MAE GERI (may ker-rey)	FRONT KICK
YOKO GERI (yo-ko ker-rey)	SIDE KICK
MAWASHI GERI (ma-wash-ee ker-rey)	ROUNDHOUSE KICK
USHIRO GERI (you-she-row ker-rey)	BACK KICK
YOKO UKEMI (yo-ko you-key-me)	SIDE BREAKFALL
JODAN JUJI UKE (jo-dan jew-jee oo-key)	RISING CROSSBLOCK
GEDAN JUJI UKE (gay-den jew-jee oo-key)	DOWNWARD CROSSBLOCK
SHUTO UKE (shew-toe oo-key)	KNIFE HAND BLOCK

TEISHO UKE (tay-shoe oo-key)	PALM HEEL
KO KUTSU DACHI (ko koo-t-sue ta-chi)	BACK STANCE
NEKO ASHI DACHI (knee-ko ash-ee ta-chi)	CAT STANCE
SHUTO UCHI (shew-toe oo-chi)	KNIFE HAND ATTACK
URAKEN UCHI (oo-rake-en oo-chi)	BACK FIST
TETSUI UCHI (tet-sue oo-chi)	HAMMER FIST
MAE GERI (may ker-ee)	FRONT LEG FRONT KICK
YOKO GERI (yo-ko ker-ree)	CLOSE QUARTER SIDE KICK
MAWASHI GERI (ma-wash-ee ker-ee)	ROUNDHOUSE KICK OFF FRONT LEG
USHIRO MAWASHI GERI (you-she-row ma-wash-ee ker-ree)	REVERSE ROUNDHOUSE KICK
JEMPO KAITEN (jen-po kay-ten)	FOREWARDS ROLL
USHIRO KAITEN (you-she-row kay-ten)	BACKWARDS ROLL
MAE UKEMI (may you-key-me)	FRONT BREAKFALL
KOKEN UKE (ko-can oo-key)	ARC FIST BLOCK
TEISHO UKE (tey-sho oo-key)	PALM HEEL BLOCK
EMPI UKE (em-pee oo-key)	ELBOW BLOCK
JODAN TSUKI (jo-dan sue-key)	UPPER CUT
MAWASHI TSUKI (ma-wash-ee sue-key)	ROUND HOUSE PUNCH
HAITO UKE (hate-o oo-key)	RIDGE HAND STRICK
MIGI SUKI GERI (me-gi sue-key ker-rey)	JUMPING CRESENT KICK
USHIRO MIGI SUKI GERI (you-she-row me-gi sue-key ker-rey	REVERSE JUMPING CRESENT KICK
MAE UKEMI (may you-key-me)	FRONT BREAKFALL TO STAGE 3

JEMPO KAITEN TO YOKO UKEMI (jen-po k-ai-ton to yo-ko you-key-me)	FORWARD ROLL INTO SIDE BREAKFALL
SUKI UKE (sue-key oo-key)	SCOOPING BLOCK (OUTSIDE AND INSIDE)
TEISHO UKE (tay-sho oo-key)	PALM HEAL BLOCK
NUKITE UCHI (new-kit-ay oo-chi)	STRAIGHT FINGER STRICK
TOHO UCHI (toe-ho oo-chi)	SWORD HEEL STRIKE
IPPON NUKITE (ip-on new-kit-ay)	ONE FINGER STRIKE
NIHON NUKITE (knee-on new-kit-ay)	TWO FINGER STRIKE
MOROTE JODAN AGE UKE (mo-rot-hey jo-dan ag-ee oo-key)	REINFORCED RISING BLOCK
MOROTE SOTE UKE (mo-rot-hey so-toe oo-key)	REINFORCED OUTSIDE FOREARM BLOCK
MOROTE GYAKU SOTO UKE (mo-rot-hey guy-a-ku so-toe oo-key)	REINFORCED REVERSED OUTSIDE FOREARM BLOCK
MOROTE UDE UKE (mo-rot-hey oo-dey oo-key)	REINFORCED INSIDE FOREARM BLOCK
MOROTE OIE TSUKI (mo-rot-hey oy soo-key)	REINFORCED LUNGE PUNCH
MOROTE GYAKU TSUKI (mo-rot-hey guy-a-ku soo-key)	REINFORCED REVERSE PUNCH
MOROTE KOKEN UCHI (mo-rot-hey coke-an oo-chi)	REINFORCED ARC FIST STRIKE
MOROTE SHUTO UCHI (mo-rot-hey shoo-tow oo-chi)	REINFORCED KNIFE HAND STRIKE
MOROTE NUKITE UCHI (mo-rot-hey new-kit-ay oo-chi)	REINFORCED STRAIGHT FINGER STRIKE

General terms.

Ai (eye) – harmony

Ai-Hanami (eye han-am-me) – same stance as opponent

Ashi-Sabaki (a-she sa-back-ee) – footwork

Atemi (a-t-hey-me) – Vulnerable Points.

Atemi-Waza (a-t-hey-me-wa-za) – Vulnerable Points Techniques

Batto (ba-toe) – Drawing a Sword.

Bokken (bo-can) – wooden replica of katana

Bu Jutsu (boo jew-jut-sue) – Martial arts

Bunkai (bun-k-eye) – Application.

Bushido (bush-ee-dow) – Way of the Samurai/ Warrior Code of Honour.

Dan (dan) – Black Belt Ranking

Do (dow) – Way of

Dojo (dow-jo) – Training Hall

Du (due) – ten

Gi or DoGi (gee or dow-gee) – Martial Arts Suit

Gishiki (gee-she-key) – Ritual

Go (g-o) – five

Hakama (hack-a-ma)– Skirt like Trousers (worn by advanced students and teachers)
Hamon (ha-m-on) – cutting edge of the sword

Hanshi (han-she) – Past Master

Hara (ha-ra) – Stomach

Hatchi (ha-chee) – eight

Henka (hen-car) – Variations

Hidari (he-da-ree) – Left

Iai (eye-ay) – Fast Sword Techniques

Iai Jutsu (eye-ay jew-t-sue) – Fast Sword Fighting

Ichi (itch-ee) – one

Itto (it-toe) – one sword

Jo (jo) – 4 foot wooden staff

Kabuto (car-boo-toe) – Helmet

Kamae (car-may) – Stance/Posture

Kata (ka-tar) – Form

Katana (ka-tan-ner) – Sword originally known as Katakiriba (ka-ta-key-ree-bar).
Ken (ken) – seeing (eyes)

Kendo (ken-dow) – Way of the sword, sport martial art

Ki (key) – Energy

Kissaki (kis-sar-key) – Tip of the Sword

Kumiuchi (kuw-me-oo-chee) – Formal name of Ju Jutsu.

Kyu Jutsu (que jew-t-sue) – Archery

Ma-ai (ma eye) – distance

Men (men) – front of the ehad

Menkyo (men-q-o) – Licence

Metsuki (met sue-key) – Focus

Migi (me-gee) – Right

Morote-Dori (mo-rot-ay do-ree) – Two Handed Wrist Grab

Ni (knee) – two

Nito (knee-toe) – Two swords

Nito-Ken (knee-toe ken) – two sword techniques

Noto (no-toe) – Sheathing the sword.

O'Hanshi (o han-she) – great past master

O'sensei (o sen-say) – Great Teacher

Obi (o-be) – belt

Okuden (o-que-den) – Master Level

Omote (o-mo-tey) – Infront

Qu (que) - nine

Rei (ray) – Bow

Rokyu (rock-oo) – six

Ryuha (roo-ha) – School

Ryuso (roo-sho) – Founder of the school

Samurai (sam-you-r-high) – Warrior or he who awaits orders

San (s-an) – three

Sei (s-ee) – four

Seiza (say-sa) – sitting posture

Seize Rei (sez-a-ray) – Kneeling Bow.

Sensei (sen-say) – one who has gone before

Seppuku (sep-poo-koo) – Ritualistic taking of ones life

Shihan (she-han) – student of the Soke who has his own students

Shikko (she-ko) - Knee Walking

Shinai (she-n-hai) – Wooden kendo sword

Shisi (she-she) – seven

Shomen-Uchi (show-man oo-chi) – Frontal strike

Soke (so-key) – Master Teacher and Founder. Also known as Soshu (so-shoe)

Taito (tay-toe) – Possession of a sword in your belt.

Tanto (tan-toe) – Dagger/knife

Tatami (ta-ta-me) – Mats, Matted Area

Tenouchi (ten –o-oo-chi) – Grip

Tori (toe-ree) – Person defending.

Tsuba (sue-bar) – Sword guard

Tsuka (sue-car) – Hilt of sword

Uchidachi (oo-chi-da-ch-ee) – Attacker.

Uke (oo-key) – Attacker

Ukenagashi (oo-ken-a-ga-she) – Deflection/Parry

Ura (you-ra) – Rear

Yoroi (yo-roy) – Armour

Zanshin (za-n-sh-in) – Awareness by spirit.